Ethnomedicine for Human and Veterinary Development

Ethnomedicine for Human and Veterinary Development

by

Dr. Ashis Kumar Ghosh
M.Sc., M.Ed., Ph.D., Diploma in Naturopathy
H.M., Habibpur Saraswati Vidyamandir
Midnapore, Paschim Medinipur-721101 (W.B.)

2009

DAYA PUBLISHING HOUSE
DELHI-110 035

ISBN 81-7035-577-X
ISBN 978-81-7035-577-9

Published by : **Daya Publishing House**
1123/74, Deva Ram Park
Tri Nagar, Delhi - 110 035
Phone: 27383999
Fax: (011) 23260116
E-mail: dayabooks@vsnl.com
Website: www.dayabooks.com

Showroom : 4760-61/23, Ansari Road,
New Delhi-110 002
Ph.: 23245578, 23244987

Laser Composed by : **Vaishnav Graphics & Systems**
New Delhi-110 055

Printed at : **Chawla Offset Printers**
Delhi - 110 052

PRINTED IN INDIA

Dedication

The author dedicates this work to the memory of late Abinash Chandra Ghosh (great grandfather, former headmaster during 1906-1914 of Rajagram S.B. Raha Institution, P.O. - Rahagram, Bankura which is previously known as Rajagram A.S. School) and to late grandfather Bhutnath Ghosh, starter of Calcutta Tram Company and to my parents.

Dr. Dulal Chandra Pal
M.Sc., Ph.D. (Cal.), F.B.S., F.E.S.,
F.I.A.T., M.N.A. Sc.
Secretary
GRAM SEVA SANGHA
P.O. Hatthuba, North 24 Parganas, W.B.
Pin 743269
Resi. : 953216-237686
953216-237167
S.T.D. : (03216)

Retd. Scientist - I
Govt. of India
Botanical Survey of India,
Indian Botanic Garden,
Howrah-711103

FOREWORD

It is known that there is a tremendous progress in development of modern medicine. Still today, medicinal plants continue to be an important source of drugs throughout the world. In fact in developed countries, there is a perceptible revival of the use of herbs in health care programmes. It is probably due to continues introduction of a large number of synthetic drugs and antibiotics by pharmaceutical companies resulted in wide spread Toxicity. Today more than 25 per cent of the formulations contain plant products. These has also been considerable increase in the sale of herbal teas and health foods. People in general are now prefer to use natural products.

Plants as source of medicine are much more important for developing countries like India. About 85 percent of the people are still dependent on traditional systems of medicine, which derives more than 90 per cent of the medicaments from higher plants.

In this perspective, unwritten and undocated tribal system of medicine has tremendous potentialities in new sources of raw materials for development of new drugs both for human and veterinary care.

Practically there is no book on this subject hence the present book entitled "Ethnomedicine for Human and Veterinary Development" written by Dr. Ashis Kumar Ghosh will be a valuable tool in the hand of students and scientists in the areas of botany, pharmacology, chemistry and pharmaceutical industries.

Dr. Dulal Chandra Pal
Retd. Scientist-1,
Govt. of India

ACKNOWLEDGEMENT

I am privileged to record my gratitude to Prof. Pranesh Banerjee, Ghatal; Prof. Bimal Das, Kharagpur; Prof. Aloke Bhattacharya, V.U.; Prof. Shyamapada Pal, V.U.; Dr. Satyahari De, IIT, Kharagpur; Asoke Nayek (H.M.); Prof. D.P. Kushari, B.U., for their keen interest in this work. My sincere thank is also due to my colleagues and M.C. Members of Saraswati Vidyamandir for their encouragement. In the preparation of this book I have received valuable suggestions and generous help from the following persons.

Dr. Madhup De, A.I. (S.E.), Paschim Medinipur; Syed Nurus Salam, D.I. (S.E.), Paschim Medinipur; Shankari Harh, D.P.O., Bankura; Dr. Prafulla Manna, Biman Gupta, Joint Secretary, District Library, Paschim Medinipur; Sudip Bej, Demonstrator, District Computer Centre, Paschim Medinipur; Aparesh Bhattacharya, District Secretary, ABTA, Medinipur; Dr. D.C.Pal, Sr. Scientist, B.S.I. Calcutta; Prof. S.D.Mishra, BARC, Mumbai; Asim Pal, A.D.I., Paschim Medinipur; Prof. Subhendu Mukherjee, C.U.; Prof. A.K. Biswas, Bishnupur; Tara Shankar Biswas, Working Secretary (Edn.), Paschim Medinipur; Nisith Das, Secretary of Sabyasachi Patrika, Paschim Medinipur.

Author wants to express his thanks to Sarathi Maity (S.I.), Biplab Ghosh and Soma Ghosh for the patience shown by them during the preparation of the manuscript. Thank is also due to all staff of the D.I. Office for their encouragement.

Dr. Ashis Kumar Ghosh

PREFACE

Medicinal plants were known to the early civilization. Tribes are using a lot of plants as drugs to curing diseases or to relieve physical disorders since the time immemorial. During 5000-4000 B.C many medicinal plants were in use in China. The use of various plants as medicines can also be obtained from the earliest literature written in Sanskrit, Greek, Hebrew etc. The Assyrians, Babyloniana, Bebrewas and Egyptians know many medicinal plants in about 1600 B.C. The works of Greeks viz. Aristottle (384 - 322 B.C), Hippocrates (460 - 370 B.C), Pythagoras and Theophrastus (370 - 287B.C) have numerous references of many of the presents day drugs.

Practically all plants are medicinal according to Jeebak (disciple of Atreya, Rajbaidya of Bimbisar) but several thousands plants have been used for medicinal properties by aboriginals and native people either by beneficial effects or harmful effects. At present medical science has paid great attention to the study of Ethnomedicine. The longest established uses of plants in remedy of ailments (both in human and animals) are widely practiced and the importance of the subject is well recognized. In recognition of the importance in basic and applied areas of the subject, many universities have been included in undergraduate and post graduate courses. The commercial uses of the medicinal plants are becoming increasingly popular. The motivation behind writing the present book was to place an introductory tent for both students and scholars including laboratories for commercial purposes.

The research work incorporated in the book has been carried out by thorough survey in remote villages of south bengal during the period from 1993 to 2002 by DR. A.K. Ghosh and the Coworkers. Some of the works has already been published in different reputed books.

1. Ethnobotany and Medicinal plants of Indian Sub-continent by J.K. Maheshwari. M/S ADVANCE BOOKS, Rajasthan.
2. Recent progress in medicinal plants, Vol. 1, By V.K. Singh *et al.* SCI TECH Pub., U.S.A and Journals of India and abroad. The contents of the book have been presented in different titles. To get a clear picture about the theme of survey titles have been enlisted appropriately under the following sub-headings :-

   1. Beneficial - For human purposes.
      For veterinary purposes.
   2. Inhibitory

Uses of medicinal herbs by tribals have also been discussed in detail.

I hope the book shall prove useful to the research scholars, teachers, students, doctors and laboratories alike.

Rathayatra, **Dr. A.K. Ghosh**

CONTENTS

1 Introduction

The primitive men have used different plant parts as therapeutical agents for remedial measures. The plants were wild and it is easy to procure them. As the recording systems were not known at that time, the methods used by them were unknown. From Rig veds, the oldest book where creative properties of some drugs were recorded, the co-existance of disease, death and medicines were observed. The sufferings and cure were intimately associated with religion, myth and magic. The work of Charaka and Sushruta, the Buddhist missionaries, the invasion of Alexander and the rise of Muhammadanism, brought a new era in medicinal practice of India. During the Christian period, the knowledge regarding indigenous drugs has been raised.

Now a days there are about 2000 drugs used in India and 1500 out of them are of plant origin. The publication of Pharmacopoeia of Bengal of '0' Shaughnessy (Professor of chemistry at Medical College, Calcutta) and Wallich (in-charge of Botanical Garden, Calcutta) gave a fresh stimulus to the study of indigenous drugs (1844). Later K.R. Kritikar and B.D. Basu (1918) wrote book on Indian Medicinal Plants, R.N. Chopra and his students presented the poisonous plants of India.

The knowledge that has descended through incomplete records through oral folklore and other unknown sources, was neglected by doctors in India. The development of biomedical practices find important steps to modern medical therapy and might be examplified by the neglected field of ethnomedicine.

From the present study it is revealed that the tribal people of Bengal have herbal treatment for common ailments and diseases.

Not only this it is also found that more the number of species for any disorder more prevalent the ailment or diseases is. Thus, the common disorders are skin diseases and injuries, headache, body ache & fever, respiratory troubles, rheumatism, diabetes, gastro-intestinal and reproductive abnormalities etc. In this direction every one should be given education so that every individual citizen can make a contribution towards protection of their own health through conservation of our own indigenous ethnomedicines which have no side effect. The young minds who attend schools and colleges, future thinkers, policy-makers and responsible citizens, need to develop appreciation towards native medicinal plants conservation.

India is a land of great natural biodiversity and one of the world's 12 megadiversity countries and a miniature form of the world. It embraces mangrove swamps of Sundarbans, rain forests of Western Ghats, coral reefs of Lakshwadweep, wetlands of Bharatpur, hot desert of Rajasthan and cold one of Ladakh. So there is a vast scope to earn foreign money by proper utilization of our indigenous ethnomedicine. The problems of biodiversity and environmental degradation call for more than scientific and technological solution. They require the re-establishment of traditional resources alongwith environmental ethics, values and sacredness of nature. The age old philosophy of co-existence is not only merely for co-existance of human beings, but it is in fact a basic premise of all living creatures and of harmony within the cosmos. The delicate balance of nature has to be restored. The balance of 5 basis elements - The Panchtatva - Air, Water, Fire, The Earth and The Sky has to be restored - Awakening to the beauty of the future through Environmental Awareness programme should be the slogan.

2 BENEFICIAL

2.1 FOR HUMAN PURPOSES

2.1.1 Ethnomedicine in Bankura District, West Bengal

Abstract

This work brings into the herbal medicines used by the tribals of Bankura District, West Bengal effective against certain common ailments. This information on further proving could enrich the present day therapeutic practice.

Bankura is one of the main tribal districts of West Bengal. The district is mostly inhabited by Santals, Oraons, Koras, Bhumijs, Mechs, Mahalis and Mundas. These men in their own unique way apply herbal medicines to encounter various diseases. The indigenous system of medicine in Bankura has almost remained unearthed. Except for a report from Chowdhury *et al.*[3] The present work is an outcome of five years field studies involving collection of data from the knowledgeable local informants on medicinal plants, their use, processing, dosage etc. for particular ailment. Voucher specimens have been collected during field trips for preservation.

The plants, their local names, parts used and the methods of application have been tabulated as detailed below against various ailments.

2.1.2 Notes on Lodha Medicine in Midnapur District West Bengal, India

This paper provides a brief account of 40 plants associated with herbal remedies among the Lodhas, a tribe of Midnapur district, West Bengal, India. Reports from informants were obtained during

Table 2.1.1

Ailment	*Local name*	*Botanical name*	*Part used*	*How medicine prepared*	*How used*
Hyperacidity and indigestion	a)Muthaghas	*Cyperus rotundus* (Cyperaceae)	Leaf	Ingredients (a+b+c) are crushed and mixed with rock salt.	One spoonful of the mixture twice daily as an antacid and stomachic.
	b) Kalojira	*Nigella sativa* (Ranunculaceae)	Cremocarp		
	c)Anantamul	*Hemidesmus indicus* (Asclepiadaceae)	Leaf		
Dyspepsia	a) Tulsi b) Pan	*Ocimum basilicum* (Labiatae) *Piper betle* (Piperaceae)	Leaf	Juice is extracted (a+b).	Two spoonful thrice daily.
Gastric Ulcer	Arjun	*Terminalia arjuna* (Combretaceae)	Bark of stem	Dust of the bark is boiled in cow milk.	Taken thrice daily till recovery.
Constipation	Jam	*Syzygium jambos* (Myrtaceae)	Leaf	No special preparation.	Chewed and eaten as purgative.
Pyorrhoea	a) Kantikel	*Solanum xanthocarpum* (Solanaceae)	Seeds	– do –	Smoked in earthen pipes.
	b) Narikel	*Cocos nucifera* (Palmae)	Root	It is burnt into ash which is combined with little amount of alum and camphor.	Used as tooth powder.
Swollen gum	Jainti	*Sesbania aegyptiaca* *S. sesban* (Papilionaceae)	Leaves	Leaves are warmed.	Warm leaves locally applied for fermentation.

contd...

Table 2.1.1 – *contd...*

Ailment	*Local name*	*Botanical name*	*Part used*	*How medicine prepared*	*How used*
Epistaxis	Akanda	*Calotropis procera* (Asclepiadaceae)	Stem	Cut into pieces and dried.	Inhalation of the smoke proves styptic.
Loss of hair	a) Am	*Mangifera indica* (Anacardiaceae)	Seeds	Immersed in water for overnight	Leachate locally applied as hair vitaliser.
	b) Bichuti	*Tragia involucrata* (Euphorbiaceae)	Flowers	Juice is extracted	Externally applied on the scalp as hair vitaliser.
Premature greying of hair	Karabi	*Nerium indicum* (Apocynaceae)	Bark of root	Bark decoction is prepared in milk.	Locally applied as hair vitaliser.
Dandruff	a) Am	Mangifera indica	Seeds	Ingredients (a+b) are crushed into a paste with milk.	Locally applied.
	b) Haritaki	*Terminalia chebula*	Fruits		
Athlete's foot Tinea pedis	Haritaki	*Terminalia chebula* (Combretaceae)	Fruits	Powdered into a paste	Locally applied.
Sepsis of nail	Am	*Mangifera indica*	Bark exudates	The sap is collected after poking the tree trunk.	Locally applied.
Burn	Chotra	*Lantana camara* (Verbenaceae)	Roots	Decoction of root is mixed with burnt mustard oil.	Locally applied.

contd...

Table 2.1.1 – *contd...*

Ailment	***Local name***	***Botanical name***	***Part used***	***How medicine prepared***	***How used***
Muscular pain	Kunch	*Abrus precatorius* (Papilionaceae)	Leaves	Crushed into a paste.	Externally applied as balm.
Goiter	Ghetu	*Clerodendrum indicum* (Verbenaceae)	Root	Root crushed with raw rice into a paste.	Locally applied.
Arthritis	Kumarika	*Smilax macrophylla* (Liliaceae)	Root	Root paste is boiled in 'ghee' (prepared from cow milk).	Rubbed locally.
Sprain	Ledachul	*Litsea sebifera* (Lauraceae)	Bark	Bark is powdered	Externally applied as balm.
Wound	a) Khair	*Acacia catechu* (Mimosaceae)	Tannin from bark	It is dissolved in water.	Locally applied as vulnerary
Anti tumour; Conjunctivitis	Mussaenda	*Mussanda pubescence* (Rubiaceae)	Sepal	Juice is extracted	-do-
	b) Jam	*Syzygium jambos*	Leaf	Juice is extracted	-do-
	c) Aswatha	*Ficus religiosa* (Moraceae)	Stem bark	Pounded into dust.	-do-
Scanty red urine	Satamuli	*Asparagus racemosus* (Liliaceae)	Root	Root crushed with sugar candy and a soft drink is prepared	Drunk

field studies. The data were compared with information obtained from some other tribal societies like the Santals and Oraons inhabiting neighbouring regions. The Lodhas have had a rich herbal folklore, but this is fading due to increasing acculturation and depletion of plant cover.

The Lodhas are the predominant tribe in Midnapur district of West Bengal, India. The district is in the south western corner of the state (between 21° 36'40" and 20° 56'40" N. and 86° 35'22" and 88° 31" 30"E). Its area is 13,000 Km^2; Woodlands cover about 1700 Km^2. The Lodhas (number about 12,000) inhabit the northwestern part of the district.

Materials and Methods

Field studies, including collections of information and voucher specimens, were made. Standard field and ethnobotanical methods were followed (Jain 1965; Jain and Rao 1976).

The principal sources of information were the older women, especially the midwives (dhai) and the older men (called baids) women talked freely about remedies for common ailments like cold, cough, fever, toothache, stomach pain and headache. They were secretive about disorders among women like matters of fertility, contraception and venereal diseases; taboos on sharing this knowledge also contributed to their reluctance to talk. Men freely accompanied the authors to the forest to collect plants. Men had no hesitation in giving information about the problems of both males and females. Diagnosis appeared to be based on experience and narration of symptoms.

Voucher specimens were prepared and are housed in the Central National Herbarium.

Information was gathered from literature also on the ethnobotany of Santals and Oraons of neighbouring areas for comparison.

Observations

The most common (and reportedly effective) methods of preparing medicines is to make an infusion by boiling the fresh or dried plant (either singly or in combination) in some cases the plant material was reported to be pounded and made into a paste. The quantity of the material used was mostly specified. Different informants gave the same method regarding use or processing a pinch of salt was a common additive to all medicines.

Lodhas believe that plants can provide remedies for most of their ailments.

Some species have restricted use; others quite wide use, in medicine. The data gathered among the Lodhas were compared with known uses of those species as recorded in Perry's (1980) work. It was found that several uses do not seem to have been recorded in Porry or in important published literature on the subject in India (Bodding 1927; Chopra et al. 1956, 1969; Jain 1968; Wealth of India 1948-1976).

The Lodhas have certain beliefs or taboos about plants. (1) Plants with latex have medicinal value. (2) Green plants before flowering are more effective than dried plants. (3) Roots are considered more effective than aerial parts. (4) Plants should not be collected for medicinal purposes in the afternoon or mid-day. (5) The medicine is more effective for the Lodhas if long pepper *(Piper longum L.)* is added and for the non-Lodha tribals if black pepper *(Piper nigrum L.)* is added. The number to be added is also significant. The Lodhas add 3 to 7 fruits of long peppers; the Santals and others generally 5, 9 or 11 black peppers. These numbers are believed to have magical powers. (6) Bark should be taken from that side of the plant on which the rising sun shines, i.e., the east. (7) Violation of any taboo can make the medicine ineffective.

We neither affirm nor deny the efficacy of any medicinal plant we included in this paper.

The Medicinal Plants

In the following account the plants are arranged alphabetically by generic name, then by specific epithet. The data are presented in this order; botanical name/name of the family/flowering period (if this datum is available)/local name is single quotation marks and as narrated by the Lodhas/name of collector and collection number in italic type/brief description and medicinal uses among the Lodhas, and some comparative notes with the Santals. Oraons and some other tribals. The medicinal uses we believe to be unique to India are marked with an asterisk.

1. *Abrus precatorius L.*/Leguminosae/Jul-Nov/Pal 3/Twining shrubs common in district/Lodha women make a paste of roots of white-seeded plants with long pepper (3:1) and take twice a day for white discharge. They eat the paste of three roots with ripe banana for promoting conception*. They take paste of root bark (about 5 g) in fever.* Santals apply paste of leaves (20-30) with limewater on swelling of glands. In Indonesia, leaves are applied on swollen tonsils (Ferry 1980). Oraons apply juice of fresh leaves on scabies* In China, seeds were used in malaria.

2. *Acacia farnesiana Willd.*/Leguminosae/Aug-Feb 'borangadaru' Pal 5/Small tree in open places throughout western part of district/Lodhas take decoction of stem bark for malaria * For contraception, women take powder of root around waist to avoid conception. Oraons believe that the plants act as repellant to rodents and snakes.* Juice of bark useful in stomach pain (Jain 1981).

3. *Achyranthes aspera L.*/Amaranthaceae/Oct-Jan/'rechari'/Pal 1/Undershurb., common weed/Lodhas take paste of plants with long pepper (2:1) for bite of mad dogs.* Tirbals of Tamilnadu use the plant for malarial fever.* People of Himalayas use the plant for leucoderma. Asurs of Bihar give decoction of plant to women after childbirth (Jain 1981). In China, decoction of root is given to bring on labor and stop acute haemorrhage (Perry 1980).

4. *Alternanthera ficoides* (L.) R. Br/Amaranthaceae/Sept-Dec/'Jal-sachiba'/Pal 2/Herb abundant in moist places/Lodha women take infusion of this plant for burning sensation in urination.* They apply asafoetida on a small piece of this plant and leave overnight in vagina as suppository for abortion.

5. *Amaranthus spinosus L.*/Amaranthaceae/'achpar-ba', Janum leper-ara'/Pal 4/An abundant weed/Lodhas smoke powder of dry roots for hallucination. Eating paste of root can cause temporary insanity.* Santals apply paste of roots on bubos in the Malay Peninsula, Paste of leaves is applied on wounds (Perry 1980).

6. *Artemisia nilagirica* (Clarke) Pamp/Compositae/Sept-Dec/'ote-palandu'/Pal 6/Shrub, also planted in Lodhas hut/

Smoke of burning dry leaves induces sleep. Its sedative property is known in southeastern Asia (Perry 1980). Santals apply leaf oil as local anesthesia.* Oraons smoke dry leaves for hallucination.* Mompas of Arunachal Pradesh apply decoction of leaves on sores. Garos of Meghalaya use the plant as remedy for asthma (Jain 1981). These uses are known in other regions of southeastern Asia (Perry 1980).

7. *Catharanthus roseus* (L.) G. Don/Apocynaceae/'Simjenga-ba'/Pal - 10/Undershrub. Cultivated; occurs as escape, or weed / Lodhas take a drop of milky juice in a cup of water in blood dysentery and give docoction of leaves to babies in griping pain. Santals apply latex on scabies.* Oraons give a drop of latex to women as galactogogue.*

8. *Coix lacryma-job L.*/Gramineae/Aug-Nov/bakri-horeng' Pal 7/ Herb; occurs in marshy places/ Lodha women take decoction of beads for menorrhagea.* Santals take decoction of seeds for thirst, dysentery, and puerperal fever (Jain and Banerjee 1974; Jain and Tarafdar 1970).* Oraons add paste of roots in country liquor to make it strong.

9. *Cyperus compressus L.*/Cyperaceae/'garajmut' Pal 9/ Herb, grows as weed/Lodhas boil the roots to the chickenpox patients.* Santals make tea from this for cold and cough.* Oraons apply boiled roots in mustard oil on septic wounds.

10. *Hemarthria compressa* (L.f) R.Br./Gramineae May-Sept/ 'Pansheru', gogyatasad' / Pal 11/Herb ; a weed in moist places/Lodhas give decoction of grass with a pinch of common salt (2:1) to improve appetite in children* Santals apply paste of roots in dyspepsia.

11. *Heteropogon contortus* (L.) P. Beauv, ex Roam, et Schult/ Gramineae/Mar-Jan/'sir-ka-tasad'Pal 8/Common grass/ Lodhas make ash of its grains and apply with 'Karanjo' (*Pongamia pinnata,* (L.) Merr oil (2:1) on piles. Santals apply paste of plant on bite of rabit, dogs, Jackals, and scorpions. They distil an oil from the awns and give with betel leaf in asthma*. They also use it for toothache, fever, muscle pain and dysentery (Jain and Tarafdar 1970). Victims of snakebite either chew the roots of the plant or take pounded roots with water (Jain 1981).

12. *Hibiscus vitifolius* L./Malvaceae/Jun Dec/'ilip-ara'/Pal 17/ Shrub, growing wild in forests of district/For contraception, Lodha women take decoction of roots with 'Mahul' (Madhuca) liquor and a pinch of common salt (1:2:1) twice daily for 7 d at the end of menstruation.* Santals apply / powder of root bark to hair for killing lice. Oraons apply paste of stem bark on bone fracture.

13. *Holoptelea integrifolia* (Roxb.) Planch. Ulmaceae/Jan-Mar/ 'chorla-daru'/Pal 13/Tree, wild in forests: planted on roadsides/Lodhas apply sap of twig on ringworm * Santals make paste of stem bark with ginger (2:1) and apply on bone fracture.* Oraons use seed oil for rheumatism. In Burma, bark is used for rheumatism (Perry 1980).

14. *Imperata cylindrica* (L.) P.Beauv/Gramineae/Feb-Jun/ 'cherotasad', 'huringchiru'/Pal 12/Tall grass all through the district / Lodhas pound the stolons with long pepper (2:1) and give for enlarged spleen and liver in children.* Santals use roots for fumigation on piles; such use also reported from Indochina (Perry 1980). Oraons take decoction of stolons as tonic in fever * Kols of Bihar use roots in fermentation of rice beer. Tribals of Khasi and Jaintia hills in Meghalaya use the grass as antidote to snake venom (Jain 1981).

15. *Kalistroemia pubescens* (Don) Dandy/Zygophyllaceae/May-Sept/ 'gara-ba' 'bongokhuru'/Pal 44/Herb, wild in southeast region of district/ Lodhas take paste of the fruits for gout.* Oraons make paste of leaves and take for blood dysentery.

16. *Lantana camara* L./Verbenaceae/'Putus'/Pal 59/Shrub, common on roadsides/ Lodhas apply decoction of leaves for relief of itching in measles and chickenpox. Santals make a paste of the leaves and apply on boils. These uses are common in other tribes in southeastern Asia (Perry 1980).

17. *Lasia aculeata Lour*/Araceae/Sept-Feb/'Kanta-saru'/Pal 14/ Undershrub, wild in moist and marshy places/Lodha women use a preparation from leaf juice as abortifacient.* They apply powder of rhizome with lime on swelling caused by mumps.

18. *Leucaena leucocephala* (Lam) De Wit/Leguminosae/Feb-Jun/'Kak-babul daru'/Pal 63 A recent introduction in the area / Lodhas seem to have only recently discovered the use of decoction of leaves for washing wounds.* They take ash of flowers for acidity.*
19. *Marsilea minuta L.*/Marsileaceae/'susni-ba'/Pal 30/Small herb in moist places/Lodha women take/decoction of stolons for insanity. Santals take a decoction of leaves with cold water to induce sleep. Oraons women pound the plant and take for menstrual complaints.
20. *Martynia annua L.*/ Pedaliaceae/Mar-Aug/ 'gaymukhi'/Pal 78/Shrub, wild in southwestern part of district/Lodha women take paste of seed for pain caused by observation in menstrual flow.* They apply seed oil for rheumatism. Santals also give leaf juice for epilepsy. Oraons pass the fresh, viscous leaves over the hair to remove lice. They apply seed powder on wounds.
21. *Mikania cordata* (Burm.f.) Robinson/Compositae/Oct- Feb/'german-lata'/Pal 8/Exotic aggressive climber/Lodhas apply paste of leaves on forehead for headache.* Santals use decoction of plant for washing septic wounds. Oraons apply crushed leaves on fresh cuts to stop bleeding. Nagas use about 150 cc leaf sap for stomach pain and for dysentery (Jain 1981). Leaves are known to be used on itch and wounds in southeastern Asia (Perry 1980).
22. *Musa paradisiaca L.*/Musaceae/'Kela-ba'/Pal 33/Shrub mostly cultivated/Lodhas tie a young leaf on the head as diaphoretic, to induce sweating and to reduce body temperature. Santals apply paste of rhizome on burn wounds. This use is known in southeastern Asia (Perry 1980). Oraons take decoction of rhizome with pounded black peppers (2:1) for diabetes.
23. *Orthosiphon rubicundus* G.Don/Labiatae/May-Sept/'Jikipota'/Pal 25/Herb occurs in eastern part of district/Lodhas take decoction of leaves with paste of seven long peppers to remove stones in urinary bladder.* Santals use the root as fermenting agent. Oraons take root for colic pain. In some southeastern Asiatic countries leaves of other species of this genus are taken as diuretic (Perry 1980).

24. *Oryza rufipogon* Griff/Gramineae/Oct-Dec/'ban-paseraxess'/ Pal 28/Grass, growing in water throughout eastern part of district/Lodhas use the sap from internodes for eye diseases.

25. *Oxystelma secamone* (L.) Karst/Asclepiadaceae/Dec-Mar/ 'Jal Kechua'/Pal 19/ 'Twiner in marshy place'/Lodha women apply about 4-cm-long piece of medium-sized fresh root to cause abortion. They apply paste of leaves for leucoderma. In China the latex of an allied species is applied on ulcers (Perry 1980).

26. *Paspalum conjugatum* Berg./Gramineae/May-Sept/'do-sir-tasad'/Pal 21/An abundant grass/Lodhas take decoction of plant for fever. Santals apply paste of roots on boils. Oraons take boiled grains with paste of black peppers (2:1) for influenza.

27. *Paspalum scrobiculatum* L./Gramineae/May-Oct/ Jome'/Pal 49/Grass occurring wild; also cultivated/Lodhas take outer covering of dehusked grains for hallucination. Santals take decoction of roots and black peppers (2:1) with a pinch of common salt for typhoid fever.

28. *Phyllanthus debilis* Klein ex Willd/Euphorbiaceae/Jun-Aug/'amla-sir-ba'/Pal 24/Herb growns as weed in cultivated fields/Lodha women take decoction of leaves for leucorrhoea. They give paste of roots to children for griping pain and hoarseness of throat. Allied species also have this use (Perry 1980).

29. *Phyllanthus fraternus* Web./Euphorbiaceae/'Bhui-amla'/ Pal 20/Weed throughout district/Lodhas take a decoction of this plant for flu and cold. Other species of genus also known to have antifebrile property (Perry 1980). Santals and Oraons mix a paste of roots of this plant and black peppers with curd (3:1:2) and take for jaundice.

30. *Pseudopogonatherum contortum* (Brongn.) A. Camus/ Gramineae/Mar-Jun/'Pansi-tasad'/Pal 29/Lodhas make paste of roots with leaf buds of 'bhoroo'(*Gardenia gummifera* L.f.) (2:1) and apply for gonorrhoea. Santals take decoction of plant as carminative, diuretic and febrifuge.

31. *Ricinus communis* L./Euphorbiaceae/Jun-Nov/'bindi'/Pal 41/Shrub, throughout district; also planted/Lodhas take decoction of leaves with an unboiled egg for 15 d for night blindness. Santals apply leaf as poultices on boils. An oil obtained by beating and boiling the seeds in water is given to children as laxative. Oraons apply leaf juice on inflammation of gums. Tribals of Khasia and Jaintia hills of Meghalaya use paste of leaves for massage for rheumatism and body swelling.

32. *Sansevieria roxburghiana* Schult.f./Agavaceae/Aug-Nov/'soch-muki-ba'/Pal 52/Herb, wild or planted as ornamental/Lodhas take paste of rhizome with that of the root bark of 'putla' (*Croton roxburghii* Bal.) and limewater (3:2:1) as antidote for snake venom. This use reported also from other parts of southeastern Asia (Perry 1980).

33. *Scleria pergracilis* (Nees) Kunth/Cyperaceae/May-Sept/'mutha-tasad'/Pal 39/Weed in open fields throughout district/Lodhas take decoction of its rhizomes and long pepper (2:1) for stomach ulcers.* Santals give decoction of plant for foot-and-mouth disease of cattle. Plant used similarly in Indonesia (Perry 1988).

34. *Scurrula philippensis* (Cham. et Schi.) G.Don/Loranthaceae/'Mar-Jul/ 'sum'/Pal 16/Parasitic on trees/Lodhas apply paste of stem bark on cancerous wounds.* Santals make paste leaves with black pepper (2:1) and apply on swollen legs. Oraons women take decoction of stem to cure vaginal discharge.

35. *Terminalia belerica* Roxb./ Combretaceae/Mar-May/'rale-daru'/Pal 22/Tree occurs throughout the western part of district /Lodhas eat dried kernels for hallucination, the narcotic property is known in southeastern Asia (Perry 1980). Santals apply fruit pulp on leprotic wounds. Oraons take infusion of fruits for cooling effect in stomach.

36. *Themeda triandra* Forssk/Gramineae/May-Jan/'sir -tasad'/Pal 27/Common weed/Lodhas boil awns in mustard oil and apply the oil on septic wounds. In China, roots given for gonorrhoea (Perry 1980). Santals give the paste of roots and a pinch of common salt (2:1) for dyspepsia.

37. *Ventilago calyculata* Tulasne/Rhamnaceae/May-Jul/ 'Raktolohara'/Pal 26/Climber in forests or wastelands/ Lodha women use seed oil locally at bedtime as abortifacient.* Santals take decoction of stem bark and black pepper (2:1) for stomach ulcer. Oraons apply the paste of plants for pain and pus in the ear (Jain 1981). In Burma, root is applied on wounds (Perry 1980).

38. *Vicoa indica* (L.) DC./Compositae/Mar-Jan/'onrka-phula-ba'/Pal 23/Herb, throughout drier parts of district/Lodhas use 3-5 cm long piece of fresh young 'twig locally as abortifacient'.

39. *Xanthium strumarium* L./Compositae/Sept-Mar/'hur-huring-ba'/Pal 31 /Herb, wild throughout the district/ Lodhas apply seed oil for rheumatism. Similar use reported from Korea (Perry 1980). Santals take bath in leaf decoction for malarial fever. Oraons apply paste of cotyledons on cancerous wounds. Miris of Assam plains use this species in preparation of rice beer.

40. *Zephyranthes rosea* Lindi./Amaryllidaceae/Apr-Sept/'peaj-kanda-ba'/Pal 34 /Wild in southern parts of district/ Lodhas apply paste of bulbs for rheumatism. Santals apply the mucilage of the bulbs on boils. Similar use is reported from China (Perry 1980). Oraons take a decoction of leaves with sugar in tuberculosis to clear the lungs of infection.

2.1.3 Herbal Folk Medicines of Bankura District, West Bengal

Key words: Herbal folk, medicinal plants

The district of Bankura, lying between 22°46'-22°38' N and 86°36'-87°46' E parallel is one of the main tribal inhabited place of West Bengal. The principal tribals are the Bhumij, Koras, Mahali, Mech, Munda, and Santal. They have their own unique culture and life style. Indeed, they have perfected their art of healing too. Inspite of rapid urbanization, effecting remarkable changes in the social, cultural and economic spheres, the traditional art of herbal cure and health care is still popular among the tribals. This indigenous system of medicine has almost remained unexplored except for a few reports (Choudhuri *et al.*, 1982; Namhata and Mukherjee, 1988).

The present endeavour aims to record the less known medicinal uses of 20 species of angiosperms as practiced by the tribals of the district, which were ascertained following a thorough screening of the literature (Chopra *et al.*, 1956; 1958 and 1969; Kirtikar and Basu 1975; Mudgal, 1987; Singh et al., 1983) in respect of the medicinal significance already documented against the respective species.

Information on the medicinal uses of plans were gathered on the basis of intensive field surveys in the tribal inhabited localities of the district, interrogation of folk doctors and knowledgeable local informants in respect of each herbal receipe and personal experience. Voucher specimens have been collected, identified and preserved in the herbarium of R.N.L. Khan Women's College, Midnapur. They are as follows :

Acacia nilotica (L) Delile ssp. *arabica, indica* (Benth.) Brenan (Mimosaceae) 'Babla'. A paste of the leaf is locally applied to cure infection of Athelete's foot, *Tinea pedis.*

Achyranthes aspera L. (Amaranthaceae) 'Apang'. A lukewarm of the root paste in 'ghee' containing 2-3 pulverized grains of black pepper is orally administered as an antidote to snakebite.

Adhatoda vasica Medic (Acanthaceae) 'Basok'. (a) Local application of fresh juice is advised as an antidote to sting by wasp. (b) A regular drinking of the decoction of the leaves serves as a prophylexis against chicken-pox.

Aegle marmelos (L.) Corr. (Rutaceae) 'Bael'. A few pieces of root bark alongwith a cupful of cow's milk is orally administered as a sedative.

Annona reticulata L. (Annonaceae) 'Ata'. A warm poultice of the leaf is locally applied for alleviating muscular pain and swelling.

Bacopa monnieri (L.) Wettestein (Scrophulariaceae) 'Brahami'. Two spoonful mixture of the plant juice in a cupful of cow's milk is drunk as a remedy for spermatorrhoea.

Basella alba L. (Basellaceae) 'Pui'. Two spoonful mixture of the leaf juice in a cupful of goat's milk is claimed to be a remedy for whooping cough.

Cocos nucifera L. (Palmae) 'Narikel' 'Narkol' . Fresh juice of root is locally applied to check loosening of teeth.

Cynodon dactylon (L) Pers. Gramineae 'Durba ghas'. A mixture of the paste of the whole plant prepared with a few grains of polished rice is claimed to overcome impotence in female.

Cyperus rotundus L. (Cyperaceae) 'Mutha ghas'. Freshly prepared juice of the whole plant is prescribed to overcome alcoholic intoxication.

Gossypium herbaceum L. (Malvaceae) 'Kapas', 'Tolo'. Local application of a warm leaf smeared with 'ghee' on boils hastens suppuration.

Hibiscus rosa-sinensis L. (Malvaceae) 'Jaba'. One spoonful of the mixture of 2-3 flower buds of *Hibiscus rosa-sinensis* in 5-7 g of the bark of *Cinnamomum zeylanicum* is orally given for regularizing menstruation.

Ipomoea aquatica Forsk. (Convolvulaceae) 'Kolmi'. A local application of the lukewarm paste of whole plant is prescribed as a remedy for retrocial abscess.

Lagenaria siceraria (Mollina) Standley (Cucurbitaceae) 'Lau'. Pulp of the green fruit is to be smeared for treatment of freckles.

Mangifera indica L. (Anacardiaceae) 'Aam'. (a) Chewing the tender leaves prevents loosening of teeth. (b) A 1 : 1 mixture of the gum from the stem bark of *Mangifera indica* and *Shorea robusta* is locally applied for curing cracks of feet in winter.

Moringa oleifera Lamk. (Moringaceae) "Sajina". Oil from seed locally rubbed for relief against gout.

Nyctanthes arbor-tristis L. (Oleaceae) 'Siuli'. A decoction of a few green seeds in coconut oil (1:3) is massaged on the scalp to remove dandruff.

Ocimum basilicum L. (Labiatae) 'Tulsi' A regular intake of 2-3 spoonful of the decoction of the leaves is given in form of soft drink as a vitaliser.

Pterospermum acerifolium Willd. (Sterculiaceae) 'Muchkunda'. Local application of poultice of the stem bark is specific for skin blemishes.

Vitex negundo L. (Verbenaceae) 'Nishinda'. The decoction of the leaf is locally applied for treating alopecia and dandruff.

2.1.4 Ethnomedicine in Bankura District, West Bengal

This work brings into focus the herbal folk medicines used by the tribals of Bankura District, West Bengal effectively against some common diseases. This information would enrich the present day therapeutic practice.

Bankura is one of the main tribal inhabited places of India. The important tribals in the district are Mundas, Santals, Oraons, Koras, Bhumijs, Mechs and Mahalis. These men remaining well below poverty level, have their own system of herbal medicine practiced since time immemorial. Human involvement in depletion of the plant resources of the nature and rapid modernization of curative systems have gradually replaced the ancient systems but tribal medicines are still prevalent. This indigenous system of medicine has almost remained unexplored except for a few reports of Chaudhuri et al (1982) Namhata and Mukherjee (1988). Namhata and Ghosh (1993). The present paper aims at preservation and dissemination of knowledge of such systems of ethnomedicine.

The present work is based on information gathered from tribal informations.

***Azadirachta indica* A. Juss.**

(Meliaceae)

Neem

a. Regular intake of fried flowers is claimed to overcome Keratomalacia.

b. Regular intake of 15 Neem leaves and 6 Bel (*Aegle marmelos*) leaves with honey serves as a prophylexis against pyorrhoea in teeth or neek cancer.

***Benincasa hispida* (Thumb) Cogn.**

(Cucurbitaceae)

'Chaul - Kumra'

Decoction of 4-5 teaspoonful of fruit juice mixed with one cupful of cow's milk and one teaspoonful of sugar is advised for cure in early stage of tuberculosis.

Cajanus cajan **(L.) Milsp.**

(Papilionaceae)

'Arhar'

A mixture of leaf juice in molasses is to be drunk for curing jaundice in early stage.

Carica papaya **L.**

(Caricaceae)

'Papaya'

a. 5-7 drops of fresh latex alongwith sugar candy is orally administered once daily to treat piles.

b. A mixture of 8-10 drops of fresh latex in one teaspoonful of lime-water and a cupful of cow's milk is to be taken one time daily in empty stomach to cure dysentery.

Centella asiatica **(L.) Urban**

(Umbelliferae)

'Thankuni'.

A lukewarm mixture of 5-6 teasponful of leaf juice in a cupful of cow's milk and a teaspoonful of honey is to be taken to check premature fall of hair.

Chenopodium album **L.**

(Chenopodiaceae)

'Bethua'

One teaspoonful of leaf juice in a cupful of freshly prepared whey is advised in hiccup.

Cinnamomum tamala **Necs**

(Lauraceae)

'Tejpata'

Two teaspoonful of decoction of 5-7 mature leaves in 3-4 cupful of water is prescribed 5-6 times a day as an expectorant.

Clerodendrum indicum **(L.) Kuntze**

(Verbenaceae)

'Ghetu'

Fresh leaf juice is locally applied on scalp to kill lice.

***Coriandrum sativum* L.**

(Umbelliferae)

'Dhoney'

Freshly prepared half a cup of juice (leaf extract) is taken in empty stomach every morning for 20-30 days 30 minutes before breakfast or any other things to cure diabetes.

***Curcuma longa* L.**

(Zingiberaceae)

'Halud'

Its paste locally applied to check blood from the cuts ends or in burn.

***Emblica officinalis* Gaertn.**

(Euphorbiaceae)

'Amlaki'

a. A mixture of Amla and Ada Powder (3:1) in water used as 'Health-drink' for treatment of bed ridden people in general weakness and in chronic disease.

b. Eating of the fruits is claimed to promote vision of person suffering from night blindness.

***Ficus carica* L.**

(Moraceae)

'Dumur'

1-2 teaspoonful of warm juice of ripe fruit is prescribed for curing anaemia.

***Ficus lacor* Buch-Ham**

(Moraceae)

'Pakur'

20-25 gm bark boiled in one litre water and taken it for 3 times for a few days. It prevents the loss of memory.

Abelmoschus esculentus L.

(*Malvaceae*)

'Dherash'

Two vertically dissected fresh fruits soaked over night in 1-2 glass cold water and drink this leachate in morning. It is very useful for diabetes and blood-cancer patient.

Mangifera indica L.

(*Anacardiaceae*)

'Aam'

Immerse 8-10 leaves for 30 minutes in cold water. These leaves are crushed and the extract taken daily to check both diabetes and blood-cancer.

Momordica charantia L.

(*Cucurbitaceae*)

'Karela'

A burnt bitter - gourd if taken daily there will be no fear for water worms and blood-cancer.

Piper betle L.

(*Piperaceae*)

'Pan'

Ingestion of 2-3 raw leaves is claimed to check diarrhoea.

Piper nigrum L.

(*Piperaceae*)

'Golmorich'

A regular drinking of lukewarm water mixed with Golmorich and edible salt serve against malaria.

Punica granatum L.

(*Punicaceae*)

'Dalim'

Fruit juice is locally used as drink to control cholesterol level.

***Zingiber officinale* Rosc.**

(Zingiberaceae)

'Ada'

Mixture of Ada and Halud (2:1) with a trace amount of edible salt in warm water is claimed to be a remedy for whooping cough.

2.1.5 Herbal Folk-remedies of Midnapore and Bankura District, West Bengal

Abstract

The work brings into focus the herbal medicines used by the tribes of both Midnapore and Bankura district very effectively against some common ailments. This information could flourish the present day therapeutic practice.

Introduction

Midnapore and Bankura are the main districts of West Bengal with large tribal population. These men are really very poor, have their own system of folk-remedies practiced from ancient time. The present reports aims at preservation and dissemination of the knowledge of such systems which have no adverse effect. Some earlier reports of folk-remedies are applicable.

Materials and Methods (Survey Methods)

The present work is an outcome of three years investigations from the veteran villagers as well as from the tribals (folk-doctors). The identity of interviewed persons are as follows :

Neul Lohar (Joypur, Bankura), Ratan Kisku (Bachurdoba, Jhargram, Midnapore), Parthasarthi Mishra (Panchal, Bankura), Amar Kisku (Chilkigarh, Midnapore).

Observation

Table 2.1.5

Folk remedies	*Local Name*	*Botanical name with family*	*Part used*	*Medicine processing*	*Dossage*
Sugar	1. Bot	*Ficus benghalensis* L. (Moraceae)	Tender leaf	Immersed 3 leaves in ½ glass water for overnight.	Leaf leachate water used as a drink in every dawn.
	2. Peyara	*Psidium guajava* (Myrtaceae)	Fruit	Immersed 4 pieces of a mature fruit in ½ glass water for overnight.	Leachate water will be drink every day.
	3. a) Neem	*Azadirachta indica* (Meliaceae)	Leaf	Regular intake of 5 neem leaves and 5 golmorich	Claimed to overcome both Blood sugar and High Blood pressure.
	b) Golmorich	*Piper nigrum* L (Piperaceae)	Fruit		
High Pressure	Sajina	*Moringa oleifera Lamk* (Moringaceae)	Leaf	Fresh leaf juice is extracted.	One spoonful juice will be fed in empty stomach daily till normal.

contd...

Table 2.1.5 – *contd...*

Folk remedies	*Local Name*	*Botanical name with family*	*Part used*	*Medicine processing*	*Dossage*
Cut wound	Shet Akanda	*Calotropis procera* (Asclepiadaceae)	Latex		Locally applied on the wound till cure.
Enuresis	Jam	*Syzygium jambos* (Myrtaceae)	Leaf	Fresh leaf juice	One spoonful juice will be fed with ghee in evening till abnormality.
Snakebite	Shet Nishinda	*Vitex negundo* L. (Verbenaceae)	Root-bark	Crushed root bark	Fed it immediately with cold water.
Habitual abortion	Durba	*Cynodon dactylon* L. (Gramineae)	Shoot	Crushed 4 shoots with 25 grains of polished rice in cold water.	Paste will be eaten once in empty stomach for a month.
Depression	Bel	*Aegle marmelos* L. (Rutaceae)	Root	Crushed the bark of root.	Fresh juice of root with a cup of milk is prescribed to induce sleep and as a remedy for weak heart.
Depression	Mehendi	*Lawsonia inermis* (Lythraceae)	Flower	Pillows are made for sleeping.	Use daily to induce sleep.
General weakness	Mosambi	*Citrus sinensis* (Rutaceae)	Fruit		Fed to patient a fruit daily.
Cataract	Bot	*Ficus benghalensis* L. (Moraceae)	Latex	Fresh latex mixed with a pinch of karpur.	Externally apply one drop once daily to the eye till cure.

2.1.6 Recognition of Traditional Medicinal Plants Resources for Different Diseases in the Student's Locally Through Introduction of Health and Environment Education Field Project

Aims and objectives

To ensuring sustainable use of the natural resources and promoting sustainable life styles for all segments of the society the field project must be included in the school curriculum. To check deforestation, disappearing plant cover and wetlands, extinction of species and tribal medicine field survey is now the essential part of school education. Field studies can influence students very actively in his community based awareness and conservation programme. This reflects students more funny and accurately the true scope of work, to caring for the needs of society that depend directly on nature for sustenance and for the fulfilment of basic human needs. Students can achieve scientific attitude such as innovative ideas, rethinking, record keeping etc.

Observations

West Midnapore is one of the largest district with the tribal population and enormous ethnomedicines. The principal tribals are Bhumij, Koras, Lodha, Mahali, Munda and Santal. They have their own system of ethnomedicine from the ancestors is now gradually being abolished. West Midnapore has almost remained unearthed except for a report from Pal (2002). The present fieldwork is an out come of 3 years efforts involving collection of data from the knowledgeable tribals.

The name of some interviewed tribals are :

1. Ratan Kisku (Bachurdoba, Jhargram)
2. Amar kisku (Chilkigarh, Midnapore)
3. Baneswar Mandi (Manikpara, Midnapore)
4. Basudeb Sui (C.K.Rd. Midnapore)

Similarly students can collect herbal drugs with the help of their biology teacher through 5 educational tours.

Conclusion

Implementing field programmes that serve as evaluation ability, observation skills, self-expression, student-tribal

Table 2.1.6

Folk remedies	***Plants used***		***Part used***	***Medicine processing***	***Dossage***
	Local Name	***Botanical name with family***			
Habitual abortion	Padma	*Nelumbium speciosum* (Nymphaeaceae)	Seeds	Crushed 4 seeds mixed with ½ glass water and a drink is prepared	Drunk once for 21 days in every morning.
Candidiasis	Mehendi	*Lawsonia inermis* (Lythraceae)	Leaf	Juice is extracted	Locally applied to the wound 2-3 times a day.
Chicken Pox-Scar	Dab	*Cocos nucifera* (Palmae)	Milk of the green coconut		Milk will be used as cream on the skin.
	Patol	*Trichosanthes dioica* (Cucurbitaceae)	Fruit	Juice extracted after burning the fruit in fire	Juice will be used like oil in skin.
Sun-Stroke	Piyaz	*Allium cepa* (Liliaceae)	Bulb		Bulb will be used as raw food which claimed as a preventive measure against sun-stroke during summer.
Hyper-acidity and indigestion	Patharkuchi	*Bryophyllum calycinum* (Crassulaceae)	Leaf	Crushed a fresh leaf with a pinch of rock salt	Two spoonful juice twice daily.

contd...

Table 2.1.6 – contd...

Folk remedies	Plants used		Part used	Medicine processing	Dossage
	Local Name	Botanical name with family			
Dysentery	Bot	*Ficus benghalensis* L. (Moraceae)	Root-cap of prop-root	2 pieces of root fried with ghee	Fed the patient once a day for 3 days.
Cholesterol	Tentul	*Tamarindus indica* L. (Caesalpinieae)	Fruit		Fed a tentul daily to reduce cholesterol.
Cut wounds	Pan	*Piper betle* L. (Piperaceae)	Petiole	Warm in fire	Locally applied to the wound thrice daily.
Spermatorrhoea	Babla	*Acacia arabica* (Mimosaceae)	Latex	10-12 gm. dried latex fried with ghee and sugar	Drunk with a glass of milk once daily for 7 days.
Menopause	Chichinga	*Trichosanthes anguina L.* (Cucurbitaceae)	Leaf with petiole	Leaf juice extracted	One spoonful twice daily for 10 days.
Bleeding	Lal-Natey	*Amaranthus tricolor* (Amaranthaceae)	Root	Extract the juice from the root	Locally applied to the cut end to check bleeding.
Memory retention	Tulsi	*Ocimum basilicum* (Labiatae)	Leaf	Extract the juice	Rubbed it as aroma therapy.

Table 2.1.6

Folk remedies	*Plants used*		*Part used*	*Medicine processing*	*Dossage*
	Local Name	*Botanical name with family*			
Dysentery	Rasun	*Allium sativum* L. (Liliaceae)	Bulb	-	1 gm of raw-rasun will be eaten twice daily in empty stomac till cure.
Madness	Chaul Kumra	*Benincasa hispida* (Cucurbitaceae)	Seed	Crushed 6 seeds and made into paste	Intake the paste with 5 drops of honey till normal.
Tinea versicolor	Shoue	*Crotalaria juncea* (Papilionaceae)	Seed	Crushed 10 seeds and made into paste	Apply it regularly for few days in the effected area. Wash it after 2 hours.
Hydrophobia	Dhutura	*Datura metal* (Solanaceae)	Ripe seed	16-40 ripe seeds will be collected (according to age vary) during the month of July.	4-10 seeds will be eaten in every morning for 4 days.
Birth control	Jaba	*Hibiscus rosa-sinensis* L. (Malvaceae)	Flower		Regular intake of a flower for first 15 days in each menstruation cycle.
Gonorrhoea (Venereal disease)	Jaljamani	*Cocculus hirsutus* (Menispermaceae)	Leaf	Crushed 3 gm. leaf with a cup of water	Fed the juice with sugar twice daily till cure.
Gall-stone & Weak-nerve	Rasun	*Allium sativum* L. (Liliaceae)	Bulb	1 gm. rasun boiled in a cup of cows milk	Drunk for 15 days.

Ailment	**Plants used**		**Parts used**	**How Medicine is prepared**	**How used**
	Local Name	**Botanical name with family**			
Blood-Coagulation	Ada	*Zingibar officinale* (Zingiberaceae)	Rhizome	Crushed and made into Paste	Locally applied on cut wound.
Bug-Killer	Muchkunda	*Pterospermum acerifolium* (Sterculiaceae)	Flower		Fresh flowers put under the bed.
Weak-heart	Dumur	*Ficus carica* (Moraceae)	Ripe fruit		2 spoonful of warm juice prescribed to cure heart.
Leucoderma	Dumur	*Ficus carica* (Moraceae)	Bark	10 gm. dry bark boiled in a glass of water	2 teaspoonful drunk for 15 days.
Loss of Memory	Tezpata	*Cinnamomum tamala* (Lauraceae)	Leaf		2 teaspoonful of decoction of 5 leaves in 3 cupful of water is prescribed for one month.
Leucoderma	Lau	*Lagenaria siceraria* (Cucurbitaceae)	Flower		Rubbed a flower regularly at the initial stage till cure.
Nephritis	Ada	*Zingiber officinale* (Zingiberaceae)	Rhizome	Extract the juice	Orally administered as claimed to be a remedy at the initial stage.

Ailment	*Plants used*		*Parts used*	*How Medicine is prepared*	*How used*
	Local Name	*Botanical name with family*			
Paralysis	Gandhal	*Paederia foetida* L. (Rubiaceae)	Leaf	Crushed 5 leaves and made into paste	Regular intake of 3 leaves as well as locally applied to paralysed organ.
Enuresis	Piaj	*Allium cepa* (Liliaceae)	Bulb	Extract the juice and mixed with a cup of cold water	Drunk the mixture once daily for few days.
Vomiting	Piaj	*Allium cepa* (Liliaceae)		Extract the juice and mixed with a cup of cold water	Fed the patient to check vomiting.
Epistaxis	Piaj	*Allium cepa* (Liliaceae)		Extract the juice	Externally applied in nostril during winter.
Abscess	Hatisur	*Heliotropium indicum* (Boraginaceae)	Leaf	Crushed the leaves and made into paste	Lukewarm paste externally applied as balm.
Candidiasis	Tentul	*Tamarindus indica* (Caesalpinieae)	Ripe fruit		Rubbed the pulp for few days.
Sprain & Jaundice	Bamunhati	*Clerodendrum indicum* (Verbenaceae)	Stem		Worn in the hand and neck.

Ailment	Plants used		Parts used	How Medicine is prepared	How used
	Local Name	Botanical name with family			
Psyzofrania	Kapas-tolo	*Gossypium herbaceum* (Malvaceae)	Root	Extract 1 teaspoonful juice	Drunk daily with a cup of cow's milk.
Weak-brain	Gulancha	*Tinospora cordifolia* (Menispermaceae)	Stem	Extract the juice	Fed it with cow's milk and sugar.
Scorpion sting	Kalojira	*Nigella sativa* L (Ranunculiaceae)	Fruit	Crushed and made into paste	Locally applied in the wound.
Eosinophilia	Joan	*Trachyspermum amni* (Umbelliferae)	Fruit	Soaked overnight in 2 cup water.	Drunk this leachate alongwith lemon-juice.
Boils	Kanthal	*Artocarpus heterophyllus* (Moraceae)	Peduncle	Crushed into paste	Suppress the boils
Abortion	Anaras	*Ananas comosus* (Bromeliaceae)	Fruit	Extract 1 glass juice mixed with salt.	Juice hastens abortion in 3-4 months pregnancy.
Milk Production	Kolmi-shak	*Ipomoea aquatica* (Convolvulaceae)	Leaf	Extract the juice	Drunk 2 spoonful daily.
Veteran weakness	Kukshima	*Blumea lacera* (Compositae)	Root	10 gm root boiled in water and then filtered	Fed it daily with lukewarm ghee.

Ailment	*Plants used*		*Parts used*	*How Medicine is prepared*	*How used*
	Local Name	*Botanical name with family*			
Anaemia	Pui	*Basella alba* L. (Basellaceae)	Fruit	Extracted the juice from the ripe fruits	A regular intake of 2-3 spoonful juice till normal.
Winterphobia	Bara elach	*Amomum subulatum* (Zingiberaceae)	Seed	Crushed 2-3 seeds and mixed with 2 cup of water.	Fed it for a few days.
Spermatorrhoea	Barboti	*Vigna catjang* (Papilionaceae)	Seed	8-10 gm fried dehusked seeds boiled in 4 cups of cow's milk	Drunk it once daily for 10 days.
Snake-bite	Shet drone	*Leucas aspera* (Labiatae)	Leaf and Stem	Extract the juice	Externally applied on the wound and fed to patient 1 spoonful per hour.
Menorrhagia	Kata notey	*Amaranthus spinosus* (Amaranthaceae)	Root	Extract the juice	Fed to patient twice daily alongwith honey.
Piles	Haritaki	*Terminalia chebula* (Combretaceae)	Fruit	Ingredients are crushed	Fed 2 gm with some amount of molasses (akh) for few days.

Ailment	Plants used		Parts used	How Medicine is prepared	How used
	Local Name	Botanical name with family			
Quicker parturition	Basak	*Adhatoda vasica* (Acanthaceae)	Root		Worn on the waist with the help of 7 threads as a waist lace till delivery.
Premature senescence	Tulsi	*Ocimum basilicum* (Labiatae)	Root		½ inch of root of tulsi and a pan taken twice daily to delay senescence.
	Pan	*Piper betle* (Piperaceae)	Leaf		
Habitual abortion	Shet Aparajita	*Clitoria ternatea* (Pepilionaceae)	Root		Worn on the waist as soon as concei-ve as a waistlace till child birth.
To get male child	Shet Akanda	*Calotropis procera* (Asclepiadaceae)	Root	Crushed a root with a cup of black cow's milk.	Fed to female at the first mens day.
	Palash	*Butea monosperma* (Papilionaceae)	Flower	Crushed a flower with a cup of black cow's milk.	Fed to wife for the first 3 days in men-strual cycle.
Quicker parturition	Shet-Apang	*Achyranthes aspera* (Amaranthaceae)	Root	Uprooted a plant by single breathing	Hanged by a white thread in waist imm-ediately when pain arise; it would facili-tate safe delivery.

Ailment	Plants used		Parts used	How Medicine is prepared	How used
	Local Name	Botanical name with family			
Aphonia	Halud	*Curcuma longa* (Zingiberaceae)	Rhizome	Grind as a dust. 2 gm dust mixed with a glass of water and a pinch of sugar.	Drunk the luke warm drink.
Night Pollution	Neem	*Azadirachta indica* (Meliaceae)	Bark of stem	Extract 25-30 drops and mixed with a cup of fresh cow's milk	Drunk for 10 days.
Antifertility	Palash	*Butea monosperma* (Papilionaceae)	Bud		Fed to female a bud daily alongwith honey for the first 21 days of each menstrual cycle.
Menorrhagia	Red Shalok	*Nymphaea nouchali* (Nymphaeaceae)	Rhizome	Crushed 5 gm and made into paste	Fed to patient once daily for 7 days to check blood.
Blindness	Sajina	*Moringa oleifera* (Moringaceae)	Leaf	Extract 2 spoonful juice	Drunk the juice once daily as a remedy for initial blindness.
Leucorrhoea	Bartaman Kala	*Musa balbisiana* (Musaceae)	Fruit	Dehusked ripe fruit mixed with a yolk of watersnail	Fed to the patient at dawn only a day.
Antifertility	Pan	*Piper betle* (Piperaceae)	Root		Ingestion of two root during ovulation period (day : 12-18).

Ailment	Plants used		Parts used	How Medicine is prepared	How used
	Local Name	Botanical name with family			
Spermatorrhoea	1. Tentul	*Tamarindus indica* (Caesalpinieae)	Seed	Ingredients (1+2) are boiled together	Fed to patient for 7 days.
	2. Mahua	*Madhuca indica* (Sapotaceae)	Flower		
Menorrhagia	Dalim	*Punica granatum* (Punicaceae)	Flower	Crushed the flower	Fed the patient along-with honey.
Elephant leg	Halud	*Curcuma longa* (Zingiberaceae)	Rhizome	Extract 1 spoonful juice and mixed with equal quantity of cow's urine.	Fed the patient along-with molasses for few days.
	Shaorah	*Streblus asper* (Moraceae)	Stem bark	Crushed in cow's urine	Fed to patient for 10 days at initial stage.
Memory loss	Nishinda	*Vitex negundo* (Verbenaceae)	Leaf	Fried 2 leaf in ghee	Regular intake claim to regain memory.
Spermatorrhoea	Haritaki	*Terminalia chebula* (Combretaceae)	Fruit		Eating of 1 raw fruit. daily to promote semen above 16 years.
Lichen	Arjun	*Terminalia arjuna* (Combretaceae)	Bark		Rubbed locally with whey
Cut-wound	Laukusita	*Eclipta alba* L. (Compositae)	Leaf	Extract the juice	Externally applied.

relationship etc. The students who have higher scientific attitude, have higher environmental and health awareness.

Educational Implications

Students learn that "In our hands now lies not only our own future but that of all other living creatures with whom we share this earth" and preserve our priceless natural heritage. Well-planned nature visits bring students nearer to nature. Development of the school herbal-garden is a good source to earn money for school-fund through co-curricular activity (eco - club, N.G.C., N.S.S). To attract non-school going adolescents movable exhibition containing medicinal plants can be arranged. Besides folk-dances, nukkad natak can be organized for them. Expected results in minimum time may be achieved by the above mentioned means.

Cost effectiveness

Students can sale natural plant products through co-operative system of medicinal plants gardening to regional drug industry. Students can engaged himself as folk doctors through self-employment programme be included in the school curriculum. It will be very helpful to develop scientific attitude among students such as (1) thinking remains always subject specific, never bear biased attitude, remain ready to accept innovative ideas (2) students collects and support scientific matter and also keeps record of it in the welfare of mankind.

Survey Method

West Midnapore is one of the largest district with ethno botanial potential and having large tribal population. Here the principal tribal are the Bhumij, Koras, Lodha, Mahali, Mech, Munda and Santal. They have their own system of ethnomedicine since the ancient time is now gradually being abolished. Students should realise the importance of wild vegetation alongwith the medicines which can be utilized for genetic manipulation also in near future. West Midnapore has almost remained unearthed except for a report from D.C. Pal (2002). The present fieldwork is an outcome of 3 years efforts.

2.1.7 Folk potential herbal drugs from Purulia, Bankura and Midnapore District

Abstract

Lesser known drugs claim on different ailments have been focused. They are very effective for their active components.

Introduction

In these districts, the demand on plant based therapeutics has increased many fold due to the growing recognition that are natural products, being non-narcotic, having no side-effects, easily available at cheap rate. These herbal drugs has little known except for a few reports. Although herbal research started in India during the period of Charaka and Jibak (Rajbaidya of Bimbisar and Lord Buddhya also a disciple of Atraya Muni in Takhyasila Viswavidyalaya) but during the last 2 decades a revolutionary efforts have been observed.

Materials & Methods (Survey Methods)

Survey was conducted during 1995 to 2002 among doctors, tribals and local communities. The discovery of new knowledge from some persons cited below :

1. Arun Ghosh (Salda, Bankura)
2. Gour Lohar (Rajsole, Joypur, Bankura)
3. Bimal Bauri and Sudhir Chatterjee (Panchal, Sonamukhi, Bankura)
4. Ratan Kisku (Bachurdova, Jhargram, Midnapore)
5. Amar Kisku (Chilkigarh, Midnapore)
6. Baneswar Mandi (Manikpara, Midnapore)
7. Basudeb Sui, (New Digha, Midnapore)
8. Sibaprasad Ghosh, (Barabazar, Purulia)

2.2 FOR VETERINARY PURPOSE

2.2.1 Herbal veterinary medicine as practiced by the tribals of Bankura district, West Bengal

This is a record of certain herbal medicines against nine common ailments of the cattle, viz., placental retention during

Table 2.1.7

Ailments	***Plants used***		***Parts used***	***How Medicine is prepared***	***How used***
	Local Name	***Botanical name with family***			
Habitual abortion	Tulsi	*Ocimum basilicum* (Labiatae)	Seed	10 gm. dry seeds soaked overnight and then crushed	Fed to the patient once daily during her mens period.
Constipation	Kala	*Musa balbisiana* (Musaceae)	Leaf	Extract ½ cup juice	Drunk the juice once daily as a remedy for constipation.
Bronchial Asthma	Kala	-do-	Leaf	-do-	Drunk the juice to get relief.
Dysmenorrhoea	Ulatkambal	*Abroma augusta* (Sterculiaceae)	Root	Crushed 10 gm. root of Ulatkambal with 2 seeds of golmarich	Fed to the patient once daily from the last week of menstruation cycle.
Irregular mens	Joan	*Trachyospermum amni* (Umbelliferae)	Seed	3 gm. seeds mixed with a cup of lukewarm cow's milk.	Regular intake for 2 times to check the abnormality.
Diabetes and Blood Sugar	Rasun	*Allium sativum* (Liliaceae)	Bulbs		One gm. fresh bulb will be eat twice daily after heavy meal for 45 days.
Dimness of vission	Hingcha	*Enhydra fluctuans* (Compositae)	Young Twigs & leaves	Extract the juice and mixed with a cup of luke warm cow's milk	Drunk it regular to improve the vision.

contd...

Table 2.1.7 – contd...

Ailments	*Plants used*		*Parts used*	*How Medicine is prepared*	*How used*
	Local Name	*Botanical name with family*			
Quicker parturition	Tentul	*Tamarindus indica* (Caesalpineae)	Root	Root should be collected from a non-flowering plants.	Tie the fresh root on hair of the patient.
	Apang	*Achyranthes aspera* (Amaranthaceae)	Root	Crushed the apang root and made into paste	Smear the paste in navel region and vagina.
Birth control	Kalo-Dhutura	*Datura stramonium* (Solanaceae)	Root	Collect the roots of black Dhutura on the 14th day of the new moon.	Wife should worn on the 14 day a cupper-amulet in the waist.
Inability	Bel	*Aegle marmelos* (Rutaceae)	Fruit	Ripe fresh fruit along with their gum	A bel will be eaten daily for one month.
Diabetes and piles	Arhar	*Cajanas cajan* (Papilionaceae)	Leaf	Extract ½ cup juice	Fed the patient once daily for 15 days in lukewarm condition.
Migraine	Ucchey	*Momordica dioica* (Cucurbitaceae)	Leaf	Extrinct fresh leaf juice	One drop of juice will be fell in the nostril and then inhale.
Sprains	Bot	*Ficus benghalensis* (Moraceae)	Bark	Crushed the bark and made into paste	Smear the lukewarm paste on the affected area as a balm.
Dyspepsia	Begun	*Solanum melongena* (Solanaceae)	Leaf	Cook the leaf to make a curry	Fed to the patient for few days.

contd...

Table 2.1.7 – contd...

Ailments	*Plants used*		*Parts used*	*How Medicine is prepared*	*How used*
	Local Name	*Botanical name with family*			
Slimness	Begun	-do-	Fruit	Burn the fruit and add a pinch of edible salt	Regular intake help to reduce fat in the body
Gout	Tentul	*Tamarindus indica* (Caesalpineae)	Leaf	Boiled the leaves in toddy and then crushed to make ointment.	Liniment the ointment twice daily till cure.
Spermatorrhoea	Kalo Tulsi	*Ocimum sanctum* (Labiatae)	Seed	50 gm seeds and 50 gm sugar candy crushed together	3 gm mixture drunk daily with a cup of lukewarm cow's milk.
Spermatorrhoea or Nocturnal emission and impotence	Kalo Tulsi	-do-	Root	Crushed the root	A regular intake claimed to cure.
Premature old age	Rasun	*Allium sativum* (Liliaceae)	Bubla	-	2 gm fresh bulb will be feed daily.
Piles	Padma	*Nelumbium speciosum* (Nymphaeaceae)	Leaf	Crushed leaf	Fed it with your luke warm rice.
High pressure	Kunch Kala	*Musa paradisiaca* (Musaceae)	Inside-stem of a plantain	Extract ½ cup juice	Drink the juice once daily till normal.
Tumour	Chalta	*Dillenia indica* (Dilleniaceae)	Leaf	Crushed the leaves	Apply on the tumour as balm.

contd...

Table 2.1.7 – *contd...*

Ailments	*Plants used*		*Parts used*	*How Medicine is prepared*	*How used*
	Local Name	*Botanical name with family*			
Alopecia areata	Jaba	*Hibiscus-rosa-sinensis* (Malvaceae)	Bud	Extract the juice as liniment and use it before half-an hour of bathe.	Follow it for 2 days in a week.
Miliaria rubra	Tejpata	*Cinnamomum tamala* (Lauraceae)	Leaf	Crushed the leaves and made into ointment	Liniment the ointment daily.
Cut wounds	Patharkuchi	*Bryophyllum calycinum* (Crassulaceae)	Leaf	Crushed the leaves and made into paste	Externally applied to check the blood and to cure wound.
Blood dysentery	Durba	*Cynodon dactylon* (Graminaceae)	Young twigs	Extract the juice (3:1) from durba and genda	½ cup juice will be drunk twice daily till cure.
	Genda	*Tagetes patula* (Compositae)	Flower	-	-
Blood dysentery	Bisalya-karani	*Polygonum recumbens* (Polygonaceae)	Young leaf	Crushed a leaf with sugar and made into ½ glass drink.	Drunk it twice daily.
Snakebite	Iswarmul	*Aristolochia indica* (Aristolochiaceae)	Leaf and Root	Crushed and made into paste	Smear the paste on wound as balm.
Filaria	Nishinda	*Vitex negundo* (Verbenaceae)	Leaf	Burn the leaves	Inhale the smoke to relief from the germ.

parturition, foot and mouth disease, cataract, constipation, worm infection, colic pain, dysentery, indigestion and louse infestation. The information has been collected from tribals of Bankura district, West Bengal.

Bankura being one of the main district of West Bengal with a large tribal population has enormous ethnobotanical potential. The important tribes in the district are Santals, Oraons, Koras, Bhumijs, Mechs, Mahalis and Mundas. They are associated with cattle as herds-men. These men remaining well below poverty level, have their own systems of herbal medicine practiced from time immemorial. Human involvement in depletion of the plant resources of the nature and rapid modernization of curative systems have gradually replaced the ancient but effective systems of tribal medicine. The present report, aims at preservation and dissemination of the knowledge of such systems of herbal medicine applicable to human patients in the same district (Chaudhuri *et al.*, 1982; Namhata and Mukherjee, 1988).

This present work is based on information gathered from tribal informants concerning common ailments of cows, buffaloes and goats in such localities as Bishnupur, Joypur, Khatra, Onda, Patrasayer, Piardoba and Ramsagar. The plants, their local names, parts used, and method of application against various ailments have been registered in table. The name of the family has been mentioned in paranthesis beneath the botanical name of each plant.

2.2.2 Herbal Veterinary Medicine from the Tribal Areas of Bankura District, West Bengal

Abstract

Ethnobotanical uses of plants in veterinary medicine by the tribals of Bankura district have been reported.

Bankura is one of the districts in West Bengal with a large tribal population. They have their own systems of herbal veterinary medicines practised since the ancient time. Due to rapid development in civilization, population and moral deterioration, a gradual depletion of the plant resources of the nature is taking place. The present paper aims at scientific cultivation and preservation of the plants as well as dissemination of the knowledge about such medicine. One should realise the importance of conserving wild

Table - 2.2.1

Ailment	Plants used		Parts used	How Medicine is prepared	How used
	Local Name	Botanical name with family			
Foot and mouth disease	1. (a) Bahera	*Terminalia chebula* Retz. (Combretaceae)	Fruit	6-8 fruits of (a) soaked overnight in cold water. To its leached	Locally applied to the wound and bandaged 4-5 times a day.
	(b) Laukusita	*Eclipta alba* (L.) Hassak (Compositae)	Root	crushed roots (5-8 gms) of (b) mixed to form a paste.	
	II. Dokta pata	*Nicotiana tabacum* L. (Solanaceae)	Cured Leaf	Crushed and soaked in cold water overnight	Locally applied.
Cataract	Bot	*Ficus benghalensis* L. (Moraceae)	Latex	Fresh extraction of latex.	Externally applied to the affected eye once daily till the opacity of the eye lens is considerably reduced.
Intestinal worms infection	a) Neem	*Azadirachta indica* A. Juss (Meliaceae)	Bark of stem	Both ingredients (1:1) made into a paste with a pinch of rock salt.	Fed 6-8 times a day and repeated till recovery.
	b) Ghetu	*Clerodendrum indicum* (L.) Kuntze (Verbenaceae)	-do-		
Constipation	Neem	*Azadirachta indica* A. juss (Meliaceae)	Bark of stem (250 gm approx.)	Decocted and then sugar candy is dissolved in it	Fed at an interval of 4-5 hours for amelioration.

contd...

Table 2.2.1 – *contd...*

Ailment	***Plants used***		***Parts used***	***How Medicine is prepared***	***How used***
	Local Name	***Botanical name with family***			
Colic pain	Bichuti	*Tragia involucrata* L. (Euphorbiaceae)	Root	Crushed and made into a paste.	Fed to the cattle alongwith its food, 4-5 times a day for relief.
Dysentery	Susni sag	*Marsilea minuta* L. (Marsileaceae)	Fresh leaves (500 gm) approx	Juice extracted and made into a soft drink.	Given 4-5 times a day.
Indigestion	Bon Kundri	*Coccinia cordifolia* (L.) Corn. (Cucurbitaceae)	Fresh leaf	Tablets are prepared from 1-2 fresh leaves, a pinch of rock salt and baking soda.	Fed 6-8 times a day.
Louse infestation	Madar	*Annona reticulata* (Annonaceae)	Fresh leaf	Juice extracted	Externally smeared all over the body after an hour or two the animal is thoroughly bathed and anointed with mustard oil. Repetition for a few days is necessary to establish cure.
Placental retention during parturition	Kanthal	*Artocarpus heterophyllus* Lam (Moraceae)	Leaf	1-2 fresh leaves smeared with raw mustard oil.	Fed to the animal.

vegetation which can be utilized for genetic manipulation also in near future. Earlier publications of Choudhuri et al. (1982); Namhata and Mukherjee (1988); Mukherjee and Namhata (1988); Namhata and Ghosh (1993); Ghosh et al; (1996) have reported the use of herbal medicines in Bankura district. This report is an addition to the above reports.

The present work is based on information collected from tribal localities of Tantipukur, Joypur, Bishnupur, Sonamukhi, Barjora, G. Ghati, Onda, Taldangra, Indpur, Mukutmonipur and Khatra villages of Bankura district. The plants their local name, parts used and method of application against various ailments have been given in table.

2.2.3 Ethno-veterinary medicine from the tribal areas of Bankura and Midnapore district, West Bengal

Abstract

Ethno-veterinary medicine preparation from different plants by the tribals as well as by local communities of Bankura and Midnapore district have been reported. All of them are really very effective and positively used by them as alternatives of allopathic medicine which have no side effect and cheaply available in both districts.

Introduction

Both Bankura and Midnapore are the main tribal inhabited districts of West Bengal. In Bankura there are 12% tribals and in Midnapore there are 10% tribals among the whole population of the respective districts. Here the tribals are Santal, Lodha, Mahali, Munda, Bhumij, Mech, Oraon, and Koras. They have their own system of enormous ethno-botanical potential would be helpful to prepare the map of medicinal plants in rardh and enrich the knowledge of pharmaceuticist. This indigenous system of medicine has little known except for a few reports.

Materials and Methods (Survey Methods)

The present survey was conducted during 1990 to 2000. Survey was made across the folk-doctors, tribals and local communities. Information collected from them at first and then applied to the cattle through 10 years to test their effectiveness.

Table - 2.2.2

Ailments / Incidents	*Plants used*		*Parts used*	*How Medicine is prepared*	*How used*
	Local Name	*Botanical name with family*			
Louse infection	Ata	*Annona reticulata* (Annonaceae)	Cotyledon	Cracked and soaked in coconut oil overnight	Externally smeared allover the body, after an hour the animal is thoroughly bathed.
Snakebite	Barachadar	*Rauvolfia canescens* (Apocynaceae)	Root	Crushed and made into a paste	Fed to the cow along with its food immediately as an antidote.
Dog bite	i. Rasun	*Allium sativum* L. (Liliaceae)	Bulb	Juice extracted and made into a soft antidote drink with milk.	Given 3-4 times a day.
	ii. (a) Bans	*Bambusa arundinacea* (Gramineae)	Root	Both ingredients (1:1) made into a paste with a cup of cow milk.	Fed immediately with grass.
	(b) Akar	*Alangium salviifolium* (Alangiaceae)	Root		
Placental retention with quicker parturition	(a) Bans	*Bambusa arundinacea* (Gramineae)	Leaf, Inflorescence	10-15 fresh leaves with 2-3 Kantal leaf.	Fed to the animal.
	(b) Kantal	*Artocarpus hedterophyllus* (Moraceae)			

contd...

Table - 2.2.2 – contd...

Ailments / Incidents	*Plants used*		*Parts used*	*How Medicine is prepared*	*How used*
	Local Name	*Botanical name with family*			
Pox	Shimool	*Bombax malabaricum* (Bombacaceae)	Seed	2 tablets are prepared from 6 seeds with a pinch of sugar candy.	Fed to the cow for 3 days serves as a prophylexis against pox.
Cataract	Dholapata	*Commelina benghalensis* (Commelinacae)	Leaf	Fresh extraction of leaf	Externally applied once daily till the opacity of the eye lens is considerably reduced.
Diarrhoea	(a) Red Shalok	*Nymphaea nouchali* (Nymphaeaceae)	Rhizome	Juice extracted mixed with curd and made into a cold drink.	Given 4-5 times a day.
	(b) Bans	*Bambusa arundinacea* (Gramineae)	Fresh Leaf		Fed to the cow.
	(c) Kanch Kala	*Musa paradisiaca* (Musaceae)	Fresh Leaf		Fed to the cattle.
Shoulder pain	Mehendi	*Lawsonia inermis* (Lythraceae)	Leaf	Made into lukewarm paste.	Locally applied to the wound 2-3 times a day.
Immunization	Babla	*Acacia arabica* (Mimosaceae)	Seed	Decoction of the seeds serves as a prophylaxis against pox, colic pain, indigestion etc.	A regular drinking of the decoction.
Asthma	Antamul	*Tylophora indica* (Asclepiadaceae)	Entire plant	Tied on the neck of cow as a necklace.	

The name of some informers in Bankura district were :

Gurupada Kisku and Ramkrishna Sahis (Danardi, Bishnupur), Gour Lohar (Rajsole, Joypur), Prafulla Mishra (Panchal, Sonamukhi), Samar Tudu (Panchal, Sonamukhi), Sunil Hembram (Sara, Raipur), and in Midnapore district were.

Bhim Kalsar (Kushpata, Ghatal), Nisith Ghosh (C.K.Rd), Pachai Kisku (Jhargram), Baneswar Mundi (Manikpara).

2.2.4 Identification, Contribution, Cultivation and Conservation of Veterinary medicinal plants in Habitat through ethno-botanical and ecological survey

Objects

Aimed at to greening the curriculum creating students and public awareness on herbal drugs (traditional medicinal plants), biodiversity and bio-piracy, thereby building a students - people's movement for self - help by rejuvenating and promoting indigenous knowledge of ethno-medicine, biodiversity and its utilization, developing field notes, tree planting, small conservation projects as well as participatory activities and make relationship between man and flora-fauna. Main aims and objectives are to spread traditional knowledge among all section of the society and to self-establishment.

Observation and Results

Survey of herbal veterinary medicines against common ailments of the cattle and birds performed through 5 educational tour by science students. The Bankura district is mostly inhabited by tribals (Santals, Bhumis, Mundas etc.) has enormous ethno botanical potential. Here people remaining well below poverty level have their own system of ethnomedicine. This indigenous system of medicine has little known except for a few reports (Mukherjee and Namhata, 1988; Ghosh, 1999, 2002).

The survey is based on discovery of knew knowledge collected from folk-doctors, tribals and local communities. Information at first collected from them and then applied actively by different students on the cattle and birds in their respective field to test their acquired knowledge. The name of some tribals folk doctors were :

Table - 2.2.3

Ailments	***Plants used***		***Parts used***	***How Medicine is prepared***	***How used***
	Local Name	***Botanical name with family***			
Slough intake (cast off skin intake of snake)	Begun	*Solanum melongena* L. (Solanaceae)	Root	Crushed one root with 3 pepper and made into paste	Fed the cow with curd once daily for 2-3 days.
Poisonous insect bite	Pathar-kuchi	*Bryophylum calycinum Salish* (Crassulaceae)	Leaf	Crushed 7 fresh leaves with 50 gm mustard oil, 25 gm molasses and 10 gm joan.	Fed the animal 2-3 times till cure.
Typhoid fever	I. Dhutura	*Datura meiel* L. (Solanaceae)	Root	Crushed a root with 5 gm of pepper and made into paste	Locally applied on head region thrice daily for 2-3 days.
	2. a. Telakucha	*Cephalandra indica Naud* (Cucurbitaceae)	Root	Ingredients (a+b+c+d in 10:2:2:2 ratio) are crushed	Fed the mixture twice daily.
	b. Swet Karabi	*Nerium indicum Mill* (Apocynaceae)	Root		
	c. Tal	*Borassus flabellifer* L. (Palmae)	Tender leaf		
	d. Kalojira	*Nigella sativa* L. (Ranunculaceae)	Fruit		
Snakebite (boas)	Sajina	*Moringa oleifera* (Moringaceae)	Dry seed	Crushed and made into paste	Fed the cow imme-diately.

contd...

Table 2.2.3 – *contd...*

Ailments	*Plants used*		*Parts used*	*How Medicine is prepared*	*How used*
	Local Name	*Botanical name with family*			
Bone fracture, joints sprain	a. Ghandhal	*Paederia foetida* L. (Rubiaceae)	Leaf	Ingredients a+b+c+d are crushed in 2:2:1:2 ratio and made into lukewarm paste.	Externally applied as balm at one day interval.
	b. Nishinda	*Vitex negundo* L. (Verbenaceae)	Leaf		
	c. Dhutura	*Datura metel* L. (Solanaceae)	Leaf		
	d. Harjora	*Cissus quadrangularis* L. (Vitaceae)	Square stem		
Placental retention during parturition	Apang	*Achyranthes aspera* L. (Amaranthaceae)	Root		Root will be hunged in tail.
Swelling throat due to cold	Mankachu	*Alocasia indica* (Araceae)	Petiole	Rotted petiole crushed and made into paste	Locally applied luke warm paste twice daily for 3 days.
Rat-bite	Sirish	*Albizia lebbeck* Benth (Mimosaceae)	Stem-bark	Crushed and made into a paste	Locally applied around the wound.
Leech-sucking	Halud	*Curcuma longa* L. (Zingiberaceae)	Rhizome	Crushed and made into dust	Locally applied to the mouth of leech and

contd...

Table 2.2.3 – *contd...*

Ailments	***Plants used***		***Parts used***	***How Medicine is prepared***	***How used***
	Local Name	***Botanical name with family***			
					helps in blood coagulation.
Milk-production	a. Tentul	*Tamarindus indica* (Caesalpinieae)	Leaf	Boiled in water with broken rich and add a pinch of rock-salt	Fed to the cattle once a day.
	b. Katanotey	*Amaranthus spinosus* (Amaranthaceae)	Entire plant		
Shoulder-wound	Koranju	*Caesalpinia crista* L. (Caesalpinieae)	Seed	Crushed and oil extracted	Oil in lukewarm condition applied externally.
Flatulence	Golmorich	*Piper nigrum* L. (Piperaceae)	Seed	Crushed 10 seeds with a pinch of rock salt and mixed in 100 gm molasses.	Fed the mixture 2-3 times a day with rice gruel.
Colic-pain	Kadam	*Anthocephalus cadamba* (Rubiaceae)	Leaf	Juice is extracted	Fed the juice with old molasses.
Snake-bite	1. Desi-Amrah	*Spondias pinnata* Kurz (Anacardiaceae)	Stem bark	-	Fed the cows.
	2. Kolmishak	*Ipomoea aquatica* Forsk (Convolvulaceae)	Entire-plant	Cut the stem according to length of the cow (mouth to tail)	Fed to the animal.

contd...

Table 2.2.3 – *contd...*

Ailments	*Plants used*		*Parts used*	*How Medicine is prepared*	*How used*
	Local Name	*Botanical name with family*			
Blood dysentery	1. Safeda	*Achras zapota* L. (Sapotaceae)	Fruit		
	2. Afing gach	*Papaver somniferum* L. (Papaveraceae)	Dried latex of unripe capsule	Ingredients of 1 and 2 are crushed with a pinch of lime earth	Fed twice for the beginning day and then doses reduced.
Loss of hair	1. Keli-Kadam	*Adina cordifolia* (Rubiaceae)	Stem-bark	Ingredients of 1+2 taken in equal amount are crushed.	Locally applied to the skin until cure.
	2. Halud	*Curcuma longa* L. (Zingiberaceae)	Rhizome		
Snakebite (Cobra venom)	Shet Lajjabati	*Mimosa pudica* (Mimosaceae)	Root	Crushed and made into paste	Fed to the cattle thrice daily.

1. Gurupada Kisku and Ramkrishna Sahis (Danardi, Bishnupur).
2. Bimal Bauri, Samar Tudu, Tulsi Pal and Manik Gore (Panchal, Sonamukhi).
3. Gour Lohar, Neul Lohar and Ajit Ghosh (Salda, Joypur).

The plants their local names, botanical names and families, parts used and method of application against various ailments have been mentioned in table.

Conclusions

To help students and social groups for acquiring awareness, knowledge, attitude, evaluation ability, observation skills, self-expression. Besides a positive attitude to conservation, social values, strong feelings of concern plants and the motivation for actively participating in its protection, improvement and against bio-piracy has been developed.

Educational Implications

Innovations of innovators, traditional uses, practices and folk remedy based on Indian raw materials of plant, animal and mineral origin and development of appropriate technologies for community benefit with special interest to the rural, urban areas.

India is one of the World's 12 mega diversity countries. A systematic study of the medicinal plants would surely generate new facts of scientific interests to students, society as well as teacher's also. Learning can be more funny if it is based on practical experience. The teacher's role is not only transforming information but rather one of being a facilitator and a resource person. Teacher's role will be to motivate the students to observe and explore the nature. Students get opportunities to join fascination field programmes and help in conserving our natural resources and heritage in a most effective manner. Humans are dependant on flora and fauna. Students should realise that (1) We are a part of nature, not superior to it (2) Aware of our natural resources (plants, animals etc.) their depletion cause threatens of human life and zoopharmacognosy.

For Indian's 60 million tribals the destruction of forests and depletion of plant alongwith animal cover has meant a cultural and social death. The forests supply these indigenous people with

Table - 2.2.4

Ailments	Plants used		Parts used	How Medicine is prepared	How used
	Local Name	Botanical name with family			
Blood coagulation	Durba	*Cynodon dactylon* (Poaceae)	Whole plant	Crushed and made into paste	Locally applied to check blood from cut end.
Pneumonia	Bahera	*Terminalia belerica* (Combretaceae)	Leaf	Burn the leaf to create smoke	
	Shaorah	*Streblus asper* (Moraceae)		-do-	
Intake of Bera pata, stagnation of water in head	Halud	*Curcuma longa* (Zingiberaceae)	Rhizome	10 gm dust mixed with a glass of water	Fed to the goat immediately for few days.
Placental retention with quicker parturition	Kukshima	*Blumea lacera* (Compositae)	Leaf		Fed to the animal.
Diarrhoea	Bans	*Bambusa arundinacea* (Graminaceae)	Leaf		Given 4-5 times a day to cow and buffalo.
Louse infestation/ bacterial infection	Halud	*Curcuma longa* (Zingiberaceae)	Rhizome	100 gm paste mixed in 5 litre water	Bathed the birds thrice daily for few days.

contd...

Table 2.2.4 – *contd...*

Ailments	***Plants used***		***Parts used***	***How Medicine is prepared***	***How used***
	Local Name	***Botanical name with family***			
Conjunctivitis	Halud	*Curcuma longa* (Zingiberaceae)	Rhizome	Crushed and made into paste and then mixed in water.	Sprayed this water in eye.
Infertility	Thankuni	*Centella asiatica* (Umbelliferae)	Leaf	Crushed the leaf with gram's dust and made into paste.	Fed to cuckoo for few days to promote fertility.
Food poison	Tentul	*Tamarindus indica* (Caesalpinieae)	Ripe fruit	Mixed the fruit pulp juice with water	Fed to the domestic animal (pig, dog etc)
	Kanch-Kala	*Musa paradisiaca* (Musaceae)	Stem	Extract 1 litre juice	Drunk the juice to hog, dog etc.
Cut wound	Chilli	*Capsicum annum* (Solanaceae)	Fruit	Crushed and made into paste	Externally applied to check blood.
Puerperal fever	a. Katanotey	*Amaranthus spinosus* (Amaranthaceae)	Root	Ingredients of a+b are crushed	Fed to the bird.
	b. Halud	*Curcuma longa* (Zingiberaceae)	Rhizome		
Colic pain	Amrul	*Oxalis corniculata* (Oxalidaceae)	Root	Crushed and made into paste	Fed to the cattle and man 4-5 times a day for relief.
Milk production	Lau	*Lagenaria siceraria* (Cucurbitaceae)	Fruit	Boiled in water with broken rice	Fed to the cattle once a day.
	Khesari	*Lathyrus sativus* L. (Papilionaceae)	Seed	Soaked in water for over night	Germinated seeds fed to the cattle once a day.

contd...

Table 2.2.4 – *contd...*

Ailments	***Plants used***		***Parts used***	***How Medicine is prepared***	***How used***
	Local Name	***Botanical name with family***			
Eczema/ shoulder wound	Dokta Pata	*Nicotiana tabacum* (Solanaceae)	Cured leaf	Soaked in water over night, then boiled and add 20 ml Mustard oil	Externally applied on the cattle wound.
Fever and cold	Chirata	*Swertia chirata* (Gentianaceae)	Stem		
	Halud	*Curcuma longa* (Zingiberaceae)	Raw rhizome	Chirata soaked in water for over night. Add this water 25 gm crushed halud and 25 gm nitre.	Drunk the mixture to the buffalo twice daily for 7 days.
	Karpur	*Cinnamomum camphora* (Lauraceae)	Leaf	Add 1 gm karpur and 2 gm nitre with 250 gm rice-liquor	Fed to the buffalo with 1.5 litre cold water.
Maggots in wounds	Karala	*Momordica charantia* (Cucurbitaceae)	Leaf	Extract juice from several leaves and add a pinch of salt	Locally applied on wound once in every morning.
Bone fractures/ Lactogenic	Keruie	*Euphorbia hirta* (Euphorbiaceae)	Leaf and Stem	Extract the juice	Fed to cattle to increase the milk during lactation period. Bubbed the juice twice daily in fracture.
Worm infestation	Somraj	*Vernonia anthelmintica* (Compositae)	Fruit	Crushed 20 gm somraj, 20 gm ada and 1 gm karpur	Fed to the goat and sheep.

contd...

Table 2.2.4 – *contd...*

Ailments	*Plants used*		*Parts used*	*How Medicine is prepared*	*How used*
	Local Name	*Botanical name with family*			
Diarrhoea	Chapakala	*Musa balbisiana* (Musaceae)	Fruit	Intact ripe fruit mixed with flattened-fried rice	Fed to the buffalo 4-5 times a day.
Milk production	Kachu	*Colocasia antiquorum* (Araceae)	Petiole	Boiled the petiole	Fed to the buffalo once a day with food.
	Mankachu	*Alocasia indica* (Araceae)	Petiole and rhizome	Boiled	Fed to the buffalo once a day with food.
	Babla	*Acacia arabica* (Mimosaceae)	Lomentum	Boiled	Fed to the buffalo once a day with food.
	Kala	*Musa balbisiana* (Musaceae)	Thor and stem	Boiled	Fed to the buffalo once a day with food.
	Tal Methi	*Borassus flabellifer* (Palmae)	Tender leaf and Methi (apex of the stem)		
Flatulence	a. Halud	*Curcuma longa* (Zingiberaceae)	Raw-Rhizome	Ingredients of a+b are crushed (1:1) and mixed with old molasses (akh 250 gm)	Fed to the goat and sheep thrice daily.
	b. Durba	*Cynodon dactylon* (Graminaceae)	Entire plant		

contd...

Table 2.2.4 – *contd...*

Ailments	*Plants used*		*Parts used*	*How Medicine is prepared*	*How used*
	Local Name	*Botanical name with family*			
Acne in tongue	Apang	*Achyranthes aspera* (Amaranthaceae)	Root	Crushed 10 grm raw rhizome of halud and 1 gm of apang root mixed with 10 ml of neem leaf juice	Rubbed the paste in goat & sheep tongue twice daily.
	Neem	*Azadirachta indica* (Meliaceae)	Leaf		
Colic Pain	Dab	*Cocos nucifera* (Palmae)	Coconut milk	250 ml milk mixed with 25 gm molasses (akh)	Drunk the mixture to goat and sheep.
Organ pain and swelling	Sajina	*Moringa oleifera* (Moringaceae)	Bark	Crushed and made into paste	Smear on the wound for 2-3 days in goat and sheep.
	Mehendi	*Lawsonia inermis* (Lythraceae)	Leaf	Made into lukewarm paste by banana leaf	Locally applied to goat and sheep.
Constipation	Haritaki	*Terminalia chebula* (Combretaceae)	Fruit	Crushed 5 fruits with one gm rock salt and mixed with a glass of water.	Fed to the horse thrice daily for amelioration.
Gout	Rice	*Oryza sativa* (Graminaceae)	Seed		Rubbed the luke warm rice gruel in the affected area of the cattle.
Foot sore in horse	Musur	*Lens culinaris* (Papilionaceae)	Cotyledon	Crushed and made into paste with water	Externally applied as vulnerary.

contd...

Table 2.2.4 – *contd...*

Ailments	*Plants used*		*Parts used*	*How Medicine is prepared*	*How used*
	Local Name	*Botanical name with family*			
Dyspepsia	Gam	*Triticum aestivum* (Graminaceae)	Seed	Crushed 1 kg and mixed with 2 litre rice-liquor	Fed to the horse once daily for 7 days.
Anorexia	Trifala a. Bahera	*Terminalia belerica* (Combretaceae)	Fruit	3 types of fruits soaked for overnight in a glass of water	Fed to the horse with a cup of cow's urine for few days.
	b. Haritaki	*T. chebula* (Combretaceae)	Fruit		
	c. Amlakhi	*Emblica officinalis* (Euphorbiaceae)			
Cough	Kata notey	*Amaranthus spinosus* (Amaranthaceae)	Spike		Fed to the horse for 3 times daily till cure.
Coldness	Kukshima	*Blumea lacera* (Compositae)	Leaf	Extract the juice	Drunk a cup of juice to the horse for 3 times.
Immunization	Chola	*Cicer arieninum* (Papilionaceae)	Seed	Both dust serves as a prophylaxis against common diseases arthritis), dyspepsia, diarrhoea etc).	A regular intake of 500 gm chola and 1 gm morich claimed to fit the horse.
	Golmorich	*Piper nigrum* (Piperaceae)	Fruit		
Cataract	Gam	*Triticum aestivum* (Poaceae)	Seed	Mixed 250 gm flour with 5 golmorich	Fed to the horse twice daily till the

contd...

Table 2.2.4 – *contd...*

Ailments	***Plants used***		***Parts used***	***How Medicine is prepared***	***How used***
	Local Name	***Botanical name with family***			
				(crushed)	opacity of the eye lens is reduced.
Dysentery	Siddhi	*Cannabis sativa* (Canabinaceae)	Leaf		Drunk the horse twice daily.
	Rai-Sarisha	*Brassica juncea* (Cruciferae)	Seed	Crushed and made into paste	Fed to the horse thrice daily
Scanty red or yellow urine	Mouri	*Foeniculum vulgare* (Umbelliferae)	Fruit	Crushed 250 gm chola, 5 gm golmorich and 20 gm mouri.	Fed to the horse once daily.
Conjunctivitis	Kolmi shak	*Ipomoea aquatica* (Convolvulaceae)	Stem	Crushed dry stem along with equal quantity of giri-soil and soaked for over-night in a cup of water.	Externally applied to the affected eye of of horse twice daily.
Thinness	Halud	*Curcuma longa* (Zingiberaceae)	Rhizome	Crushed 5 gm halud and 1 gm alum	Fed to the horse once daily during winter with food-grain.
Flatulence	Mustard oil	*Brassica campestris* (Cruciferae)	Seed	Extract the oil and mixed with soft-soap	Smear the luke-warm mixture on the belly of the horse.
	Isabgul	*Plantaqo ovata* (Plantaginaceae)	Seed coat	Crushed and made into paste	Smear on the abdo-men of the horse.
	Old pond-mud			Fresh	Externally applied as balm on belly.

contd...

Table 2.2.4 – *contd...*

Ailments	*Plants used*		*Parts used*	*How Medicine is prepared*	*How used*
	Local Name	*Botanical name with family*			
Anorexia	Hing	*Ferula asafoetida* (Umbelliferae)	Resin of root	Crushed 1 gm hing and mixed with 250 gm Chola-dust	Fed to the horse alongwith a pinch of rock-salt at dawn in empty stomach.
Weaknes	Gulancha	*Tinospora cordifolia* (Menispermaceae)	Stem	Extract 1 cup juice for horse	Drunk the juice once daily.
	Ghee				Massage the colt with ghee for 7 days after birth.
Gout with wound	1. Indigo	*Indigofera tinctoria* (Papilionaceae)	Leaf	Ingredients (1:1:1) are crushed	Fed to the horse once daily for 10 days.
	2. Pan	*Piper betle* (Piperaceae)	Leaf		
	3. Nishinda (Boan)	*Vitex negundo* (Verbenaceae)	Leaf		
Diabetes/ Glycaemies	Chola	*Cicer arietinum* (Papilionaceae)	Seed	A pinch of wax and borax will be added to food-grain.	Fed to the hrose daily for few days.
Alopecia					Rubbed the stale mop at dawn in calf.
Colic pain	Baichi	*Flacourtia indica* (Flacourtiaceae)	Root bark	Crushed (10 gm. each) into paste.	Fed to the buffalo thrice daily.

contd...

Table 2.2.4 – *contd...*

Ailments	*Plants used*		*Parts used*	*How Medicine is prepared*	*How used*
	Local Name	*Botanical name with family*			
	Indrajab	*Holarrhena antidysenterica* (Apocynaceae)	Seed		- do -
	Somraj	*Vernonia anthelmintica* (Compositae)	Seed		- do -
Gout	Monsha	*Opuntia dillenii* (Cactaceae)	Latex	Crushed sulpher, salt, nitre (25 gm. each) with 10 drops latex and required amount of stale water of hookah	Rubbed locally for few days in goat and sheep.
Worm infection	Kagzilebu	*Citrus aurantifolia* (Rutaceae)	Leaf	Extract 1 cup juice and mixed with 2 cup stale water of hookah	Drunk the buffalo with a pinch of salt in empty stomach for few days.
Conjunctivitis	Hatisur	*Heliotropium indicum* (Boraginaceae)	Leaf	Extract the juice	Apply 1 drop to eye thrice daily.
Poisonous wound	Katanotey	*Amaranthus spinosus* (Amaranthaceae)	Root	Crushed the root into paste	Smeared on the wound.
Poisonous wound	Gosap (animal)	*Varanus benghalensis*	Fat	Extract the oil	Smeared on the wound.
Gout and wound	Porcupine (animal)		Fat	Extract the oil	Smeared on the wound.

contd...

Table 2.2.4 – *contd...*

Ailments	Plants used		Parts used	How Medicine is prepared	How used
	Local Name	Botanical name with family			
Dimness of vision	Bak	*Sesbania grandiflora* (Papilionaceae)	Flower		Fed the flower to cattle alongwith food.
Constipation (acidity)	Kanch kala	*Musa paradisiaca* (Musaceae)	Leaf	Crushed the leaf and made into paste	Fed to cattle twice daily.
Bronchial asthma	Kanch kala	*Musa paradisiaca* (Musaceae)	Leaf	Crushed the leaf and made into paste	Fed to cattle twice daily.
Bone fracture	Arjun	*Terminalia arjuna* (Combretaceae)	Bark	Crushed 25 gm. bark and 5 gm. bulb into paste	Externally applied as balm once daily.
	Rasun	*Allium sativum* (Liliaceae)	Bulb		
Dysentery	Ganda	*Tagetes patula* (Compositae)	Flower	Extract a glass of juice (2:5)	Drunk the juice to cattle twice daily.
	Durba	*Cynodon dactylon* (Poaceae)	Leaf and stem		

water, fuel, fodder, fibre and food. Students must realize therefore "Conservation of plants, animals, nature and natural resources (like water, minerals) is not a luxury but a vital investment in their future to earn a lot of money.

Cost effectiveness

Biopiracy deprives Bengalee in 3 ways:

1. It creates a false claim to novelty and invention, even though the knowledge has evolved since ancient time in Bengal.
2. It divests scarce biological resources to monopoly control of corporations thus depriving local communities and indigenous practitioners (folk-doctors).
3. It creates market monopolies and excludes the original innovators for their rightful share to local national and global markets.

2.2.5 Herbs used to treat different diseases in animals

Introduction

The paper narrates a brief account of herbal veterinary medicines among the tribes of west midnapore district, West Bengal, India. Reports from different tribes are compared with the information obtained from local communities inhabiting in the district. This district is in the south-western corner of the state between 21° 36'40" and 20° 56'40" N & 86° 35'22" and 88° 31'30"E.

Materials and Methods

Informations were collected during 1995-2002. The principal sources of information were the folk-doctors and the older men. I have talked them freely about remedies for common ailments. Diagnosis reported to be based on their experience.

Observations

The tribals have certain beliefs about plants :

1. Plants should be collected for medicinal uses in the morning.
2. Roots are considered more effective compared to aerial parts.

3. Fresh plants before flowering are more effective than dried plants.
4. Plants with latex have medicinal properties.
5. Bark should be collected from the east side of the plant (specially in Arjun tree).
6. The medicine is more effective if pepper is added. Violation of the above mentioned beliefs or taboos can make the medicine ineffective.

2.2.6 Preventive health care of cattle diseases

There are various diseases of cows colt buff, buffalo's and goats caused by bacteria, viruses, parasites protozoa and other non-infectious agents. The most clinical manifestations of some of these diseases are given. The diagnosis of the diseases based only on clinical symptoms is most difficult, as many diseases resemble one another. The important clinical symptoms of common diseases have been given only to help the farmers to detect the sick animal at the earliest. In case of the serious disease problem, the farmers may take some steps, as recommended, so as to prevent deterioration in the condition of animal, till it is brought under the supervision of health specialist. It is our observations that preventive care play a very significant role and the occurrence of diseases and its seriousness can be prevented or minimized if timely preventive health care has been adopted in farming by green medicine.

"Common Diseases of Cattle."

1. Rinderpest

Symptoms : There is mild thermal reaction and diarrhoea. Ulcerative lesions appeared on inside the lower lip and gums.

2. Foot and Mouth Diseases Virus (O.A.C and Asia one type)

Symptoms : The disease is mild in adult. Vesicles on the tongue, lips, cheeks, gums, dental pad and on the skin between claws, occasional blisters on teats (nipples) and udder. Lameness is also seen in adult. Deaths have been observed in young.

Preventive care : Isolate the sick goats and vaccinate the herd at the face of outbreak. Wash the mouth of infected goat with mild disinfectants like Alum, Potassium permanganate. Apply extract of *Eclipta alba* or boroglycerine on the ulcers.

Table 2.2.5

Ailment	*Local Name*	*Botanical name with family*	*Parts used*	*How medicine is prepared*	*How used*
Diarrhoea	Satamuli	*Asparagus racemosus* (Liliaceae)	Root	Crushed the root with water	Fed the cow twice daily.
	Apang	*Achyranthes aspera* (Amaranthaceae)	Root	Crushed 1 gm root and made into paste.	Fed the cow once daily.
	Anaras	*Ananas comosus* (Bromeliaceae)	Leaf	Extract the juice	Drunk the juice twice daily.
Flatulence	Gulancha	*Tinospora cordifolia* (Menispermaceae)	Leaf and stem	Crushed and made into paste	Fed twice daily till cure.
Dog bite	Akanda	*Calotropis procera* (Asclepiadaceae)	9-flowers	Crushed flowers along with a pinch of karpur	Fed to affected animal.
	Karpur	*Cinnamomum camphora* (Lauraceae)			
	Tiger tongue	*Panthera tigris*		Tiger tongue also claimed as a preventive measure.	
Lice in wound	Swet bichuti	*Tragia involucrata* (Euphorbiaceae)	Root		A man who tie a root in the tail shall never touch the cow for 7 days.
Food poison	Iswarmul	*Aristolochia indica* (Aristolochiaceae)	Leaf	Extrct 5 ml. juice	Drunk the juice.
Lactogenic	Dherash	*Abelmoschus esculentus* (Malvaceae)	Root	Hang the root in tail after delivery to get as usual milk.	

contd...

Table 2.2.5 – *contd...*

Ailment	***Local Name***	***Botanical name with family***	***Parts used***	***How medicine is prepared***	***How used***
Foot and mouth disease	Dherash			Buried the root in cow shed.	
Castrated wound	Rasun-oil	*Allium sativum* (Liliaceae)	Bulb	Bulb boiled in mustard oil	Smear the oil in wound.
Eczema	Dokta pata	*Nicotiana tabacum* L. (Solanaceae)	Cured leaf	Crushed and soaked in cold water overnight.	Locally applied twice daily till cure.
Blood dysentery	Jam	*Syzygium cumini* (Myrtaceae)	Bark	Crushed the bark and made paste	Fed twice daily till cure.
Colic pain	Cockroach	*Periplanata americana*	Juice	Fry the animal in ghee	Fed to animal thrice daily.
Eruption	Choulmoogra oil	*Hydnocarpus kurzil* (Flacourtiaceae)	Seeds	Pressed out of the seeds	Smear the oil in skin.
Chicken pox, Diarrhoea, Blood dysentery	Boncharal	*Desmodium gyrans* (Papilionaceae)	Leaf		Fed to the cow 4 leaves thrice daily.
Swelling throat	Kanga	*Agave sisalana* (Agavaceae)	Leaf	Extract the juice	Smear the juice.
Foot and mouth disease	Apang	*Achyranthes aspera* (Amaranthaceae)	Root	Crushed 1 gm root and made into a paste	Fed the cow twice daily.
Bacillary dysentery	Bisalyakarani	*Polygonum recumbens* (Polygonaceae)	Leaf	Crushed 2-3 leaves with sugar and made into a glass of drink.	Drunk it twice till check.
Colic pain	Peyara	*Psidium guajava* (Myrtaceae)	Leaf	Crushed a man's lice with a peyara leaf	Fed to the animal thrice daily till cure.

3. Pox

Symptoms : Slight fever, congested area and vesicles appear on ear, nose and udder. After vesicles containing pus, dry crust are formed. High temperature is there, but death occurs before development of skin lesions.

Preventive care : Isolate the sick animal and daily washing the lesions with neem leaves juice or hydrogen peroxide dilute with equal part of warm water followed by antibiotic cream. Milkers hand scrubbed in non-irritant antiseptic solution.

4. Contagious Ecthyma.

Symptoms : Pustular and scabby lesions develop on the muzzle and lips.

Bronchopneumonia and gastroenteritis have been observed. Morbidity rate is very high 50-60% but mortality rate may be 5% in kids and calves.

Preventive care : To check the spread, infected beasts should be isolated. The lesions should be treated with antiseptic drugs. In generalized or systematic infection antibiotic should be given to prevent secondary bacterial complication.

5. Rabies

Symptoms: The disease develops usually after 20-60 days of bite, but not less than 10 days of bite. The animal becomes strange in behaviour and there is frothing and salivation. The animal does not eat or drink, slowly becomes paralysed and dies within 10 days of onset of disease.

Preventive care : Vaccinate soon after dog bite.

6. Johne's Disease (Mycobacterium paratuberculosis)

Symptoms : In goats loss of body weight, weakness and emaciation. Frequent diarrhoea in some adult goats. The clinical disease observed after 1-2 years of age in goats.

Preventive care : Consult the good health specialist for testing of your goats. Segregate and cull the positive goat. There is no reliable test to detect J.D. in very initial stages.

7. Brucellosis (Brucella organisms)

Symptoms : Abortion in late pregnancy is the feature of the disease, retention of placenta and metritis are common.

Preventive care : Get your animal tested for brucellosis and isolate or cull the positive animals.

8. Haemorrhagic Septicaemia (P. multocida)

Clinical Symptoms : High fever, difficult respirations, coughing and sudden death may occur.

Prevention care : Vaccination with H.S. Adjuvant vaccine is recommended before onset of rains.

9. Anthrax (Bacillus anthracis)

Symptoms : Sudden high temperature (108°F), loss of appetite and sudden death. In less peracute form, live for a day and develop bloody diarrhoea.

Preventive care : Keep the affected animal separately. Animal vaccination of goats, colt calves in endemic area is recommended. Massive doses of penicillin I/M may response. Dead animal must be buried in the ground.

10. Collibacillosis / Collisepticaemia (E. coli)

Symptoms : Under one to six months of age are commonly effected. Important symptoms are fever, diarrhoea or dysentery, loss of appetite, dryness of hair and skin coat. In later stages, temperature become subnormal.

Preventive care : Rectal swabs to have *E. coil* and sensitivity test depending upon sensitivity, does all newborns with a specific antibiotic. Darzin with neomycin, chloromycetin. Septran and quixalin bolus etc are commonly used.

11. Enterotoxaemia

Symptoms : Severe pain in the abdominal region, excitement, kids jump in the air and fell down, and sudden death is there.

Preventive care : Kids of 3 months age should be vaccinated with 2.5 ml vaccine S/C and repeated after 14 days. Annual vaccination is required.

12. Tuberculosis (Mycobacterium tuberculosis)

Symptoms: Irregular low grade fever of long duration, coughing, difficulty in respiration, anaemia, progressive emaciation and loss of body weight are the common clinical manifestations.

Preventive care : Consult good folk health specialist and get your animal tested with tuberculin and drunk the juice of chaul-kumra (*Benincasa hispida*).

13. Chlamydiosis

Symptoms : Pneumonia, sometimes diarrhoea is present in goats. The pregnant goats may also abort in early stage of gestation. In young kids arthritis is developed.

Preventive care : Treatment with penicillin is effective.

14. Mycoplasmosis (M.agalactiae. M.Capri. M.capricollum)

Symptoms : There is high rise of temperature with respiratory trouble. In some cases arthritis, mastitis in lactating goats are the usual clinical features.

Preventive care : Treatment of affected goats with tylosin or erythromycin was found to be effective in early stage. Oxytetracyclin was also effective in reducing severity of disease.

15. Mastitis (Staphylococci, Streptococci, E.coli, Mycoplasma agalactiae, M.arginini, Yeast and Fungi)

Symptoms : Fever in acute mastitis, udder is enlarged, hot painful, milk become watery, inconsistency often with flakes of blood, udder become hard, milk secretion very much reduced. In *M. agalactiae,* the affected quarter become atrophic or agalactic.

Preventive care : After washing with $KMnO_4$ solution, remove the milk carefully from the affected quarter. Introduce antibiotic 1/ mammary infusion, leave for 24 hours and repeat for 3 yrs. Get your goat tested regularly to detect subclinical mastitis.

16. Coccidiosis

Symptoms: Diarrhoea, anaemia, weakness and death is seen in coccidiosis of kids.

Preventive care : Faecal examination is needed. Sulphamezathine 0.2 gm/kg body weight. Amprosol 20% solution 100mg/ kg body weight 4-5 days are effective.

17. Verminous Pneumonia (Dictyocaulus fuilaria)

Symptoms : Respiratory trouble with persistent or severe coughing. There is usually discharge from eye and nostrils.

Preventive care : Vaccination is commonly used against *D. filaria*. Dictyciden and Diethylcarbamazine are effective.

18. Parasitic gastroenteritis (Haemonchus, Trichostrongylus, Oesophago-stomum etc.)

Symptoms : Diarrhoea severe anaemia (white eyes), emaciation and watery swelling under the jaw (Bottle Jaw) are the common symptoms.

Preventive care : Faecal examination is necessary. Nilverm ICI @ 15 mg/kg body weight or Panacur @ 5 mg/kg body weight and Thiobendazole 50 mg/kg weight should he given.

19. Liver Fluke (Faciola gigantica)

Symptoms : Diarrhoea, emaciation and oedema of throat are commonly observed.

Preventive care : Faecal examination is essential. Zanil (ICI) @ 10-15 mg/kg body weight and Distodin 20 mg/kg weight are effective.

20. Parasitic winter diarrhoea (Paramphistomiasis)

Symptoms : Occurs from October to March, loose to watery diarrhoea, bottle jaw condition is advance, clinical cases are the main features.

Preventive care : The disease is caused by immature stages. Post-mortem of the affected animal is necessary for diagnosis. Zanil @ 10-15 mg/kg and Nilzan 10-15 mg/kg body weight are very effective.

21. Tape worm (moniezia etc.)

Symptoms : Diarrhoea and constipation, segments of tape worm may be seen in the faeces.

Preventive care : Panacur @ 10 mg/kg body weight is very effective. Kamala 2-3 gm/animal is also effective.

22. Ectoparasitic Infestations (Ticks, Sucking lice)

Symptoms : Cause irritation, anaemia, ill health and transmit many diseases.

Preventive care : Regular dipping with 0.5% Seven or 0.2% Cythion at monthly interval or whenever needed. Seven dust 5% is also used for lice. Smeared the seed paste of Ata (*Annona squamosa*) for an hour and then bathed.

23. Mange (Sarcoptes, Demodatic and Psoroptes)

Symptoms : Flakey scurfy dandruff on the skin, severe itching, hairlessness develops and the skin becomes thick, hard and corrugated.

Preventive care : Skin scraping examination is essential. Clip hair and wash warm water and soap. Apply 0.5% malathion or 0.5 Seven or 0.06% Lindane as spray. Swab or dip thrice at the interval of 7 days. Diptrex ointment 1% is effective.

24. Ring worm (Fungus)

Symptoms : Inflammation of hair follicles, falling of hairs, lesions are circular on the face, shoulder, neck, eyes, irritation and rubbing, thick crusts or scales may appear.

Preventive care : After clipping hair and scrubbing with water and soap, apply acid salicylic or benzoic acid ointment 2-5% or tincture of iodine once daily till lesions heal. Smeared the paste of Dokta pata (*Nicotiana tabacum*).

25. Tympany Bloat (Acidosis due to green fodder concentrate rich in carbohydrade such as Rice, Wheat, Gwar etc.)

Symptoms : Inappetance, dullness depression, increase pulse and respiration rate are seen. Distended abdomen on left side due to dilated rumen (tight as drum). Froth comes from mouth, animal became restless, repeated lying down and die in short period.

Preventive care : Drench carefully 28 gm soda in 284 ml. of hot water. A cup of mineral oil may also relieve the condition. In acute cases removal of gas with thick needle is needed.

26. Milk fever (Low level of blood calcium)

Symptoms : Include anxiety, uncontrolled movements, staggering gait, collapse and death. It occurs with 48 hours of kidding.

Preventing care : Curing milk fever needs quick action for I/V calcium borogluconate.

27. Hydrocyanic Acid (Jwar, Baru)

Symptoms : Nervous symptoms and sudden death of the goat.

Preventive care : Blood is bright red in colour. Sodium thiosulphate 2 gm in 15 ml of water s/cut and sodium nitrite 1 gm are to be given.

28. Urea poisoning (Urea/might have been taken accidentally)

Symptoms : Severe abdominal pain, tremors, dyspnoea and bloat.

Preventive care : Vinegar or 2% acetic acid is to be given orally in repeated doses. Drink the leaf juice of Iswarmul (*Aristolochia indica*).

29. Nitrate/nitrite poisoning (Nitrate/nitrite rich fodder-maize/bajra)

Symptoms : Respiratory difficulty staggering gait, falling sudden death and urine positive for nitrate/nitrite are the usual clinical manifestations.

Preventive care : Blood become chocolate brown in colour, treat the sick goat and cattle with Vitamin. C and Methyline. Drunk the leaf juice of Iswarmul (*Aristolochia indica*).

30. Insecticides (Aldrin, Endrin, Chlordane and Dieldrin)

Symptoms : Uneasiness, dizziness and tremors, convulsions. Death from respiratory arrest during coma are the important symptoms.

Preventive care : A saline purgative may be given. To control convulsion Phenobarbital or largactil may be given. Calcium gluconate 10% may be given I/V followed by antidote. Drink the leaf juice of Iswarmul.

2.2.7 Preventive health care for cattle

The following few general points are essential to prevent calf, colt and kid mortality, particularly in an organized farm:

1. At birth ligate the umbilical cord and apply Tincture iodine for two days.
2. Soon after birth remove the membrane over the mouth, nostrils etc. and clean with dry cloth.
3. In case the calf, colt and kid does not start breathing, lift it by holding its hind legs with head downward and give a slight jerk. Repeat again till breathings starts. Compression and relaxation of chest help breathing.
4. Wash the udder with mild solution of Dettol or Potassium permanganate before feeding to the kid, calf and colt.
5. Feed colostrum @10% of the body weight three times a day for 3-4 days followed by twice a day.
6. Feed colostrum within 30 minutes or soon after birth.
7. Colostrum of step mother should not be fed.
8. Do not add antibiotic or vitamins to the colostrum and milk.

9. Separate the new born from the mother after 5-7 days after birth. Neither the new born will be refused.
10. Disinfect the calf, colt and kid pens with phenyl (10% solution) or copper sulphate (1% solution).
11. If mother is heavy milker, then remove the excess quantity of milk before feeding to the new born.
12. Provide fresh water if require.
13. Green fodder such as soft leaves, grasses may be given to the kids, colts and calves after 10 days of birth may be given.
14. Supplement milk with minerals such as iron, copper, magnesium, cobalt, zinc and salt etc. will be given.
15. To prevent coccidiosis amprosol may be given for 5-6 days.
16. Protect new born against extreme weather conditions, particularly during first 3-4 weeks of age.
17. Control the ticks and flies by spraying malathion (0.5% solution).
18. For ectoparasites, dipping calves and kids should be done in 0.5% Malathion solution. Care should be taken to prevent the entry of solution in the eyes, nose, ears or mouth.
19. Replace the soil within every 15 days and add lime to prevent over concentration of bacteria, eggs or cyst in the shed.
20. Do not keep more number of new born in a limited space.
21. For prevention of internal parasites use Nilverm, Panacur, or Thiobenda-zole.
22. At the age of 3 months, administered sub/cut multicomponent clostridial vaccine.
23. In case of sickness, isolate the new born from other healthy calves, colts, kids and consult folk doctor.
24. Do not make indiscriminate use of antibiotic and antiparasitic drugs. For any problem, consult good health specialist or folk doctor.
25. More attention will be given on herbal medicine. As it has no adverse effect.

3
INHIBITORY

3.1 Inhibitory effect of fishes exposed to some cultivated, wild plant from the Bangiya West Rardh (Bankura, Midnapore and Purulia District)

Inland aquatic ecosystem occupy a peerless status among the protein sources of the country. Due to continued rise in price of fishes, the protein crisis for human being in West Bengal have prompted to search for better fish management. West Bengal secures the top position for fish production in India and specially the village Ramsagar in Bankura district, stands first in fish spawning.

In the modern pisciculture techniques, the preparation of suitable water bodies by eradicating the unwanted fishes and other harmful aquatic flora and fauna is a prime importance. Weed management in our country is done either manually or chemically by weedicides, pesticides or piscicides. These toxic chemicals are costly, and even harmful to fish culture.

On the contrary phytotoxins act as narcotic or stupefy the fish species and other aquatic fauna, also act as organic manure after decomposition where fishery coexists in close harmony with other uses of water.

Plant derived fish toxicants cause respiratory choking, haemolysis of the gills and lower the dissolved oxygen level of water bodies. Some plant exudates cause blindness to fishes which often swimming for a while, come to rest and are easily caught by fishermen.

Phytotoxins are extensively used all over the world for eradication of unwanted fishes during prestocking pond management or during poaching (Naskar, 1986). Further the affected fishes are not harmful for human consumption.

Piscicides of plant origin such as Mahua oil cake (*Madhuca indica*), rootdust of *Derris scandens, D. trifoliata,* seed dust of *Croton tiglium, Milletia spicida, M. pachycarpa* and bark powder of *Barringtonia acutangula, B. racemosa* are in use since 1834 (Naskar and Guha Bakshi, 1987).

A few plants from 'Bangiya West Rardh' region possessing such piscicides properties are discussed. Generally plant derivates contain abrin, crotin, clerodin, cerotic, cautohoue, glycosides, kranjin, lignoceric, lindic acid, meliatin, oleic paraisine, quercetin, rotenon and saponin (Tyler *et al.* 1981). Only Mahua oil cake (plant toxicant) is used for pond management. With the rapid developed of piscicultural technique and due to short supply of pure mahua oil cake it has now become necessary to find alternative piscicides of plant origin.

Many plant in Bangiya West Rardh regions listed below possess such piscicidal properties.

Annona squamosa (Ata, Annonaceae) : Shrub growing up to 10-15' high. Found generally in village surroundings. Seeds contain anonaine (alkaloid 0.03%). Seeds are reported to be a piscicide and insecticide, the bark.is also astringent.

Achyranthes aspera (Apang, Amaranthaceae) : Annual herb, 2-3' high, leaf, root and seeds are reported to be toxic to fishery.

Cannabis sativa (Ganja, Cannabinaceae) : Erect annual undershrub, dioecious, height 7-8'. Female plant is cultivated as a narcotic and drug plants.

Opuntia dillenii (Mansa, Cactaceae) : A common xerophyte with phylloclade bearing many spines. The latex is toxic to the fishes.

Tamarindus indica (Tentul, Caesalpiniaceae) : A tall sub-evergreen tree. Occasionally planted and frequently found in forest and in village along roadsides. Seed dusts are used as toxicant for fishes. This chokes gills, effects respiration and kills the fish. Seed husk of 1800-2000 kg/hac at 1 m. depth is enough to kill the fishes. Toxic effect persists for 20-25 days.

Papaver somniferum (Afing gach, Papaveraceae) : Annual herb with large showy flowers, commonly cultivated. Opium is the dried latex or juice obtained from the unripe capsule of the plant. Crude opium contain many alkaloids. An alkaloid known as morphine is obtained from it. Opium has got narcotic to fishes.

Croton tiglium (Bheranda, Euphorbiaceae) : Plant is a small evergreen tree or shrub, rarely cultivated. Croton oil is a fatty oil obtain from the dried ripe seed, is a yellowish-brown liquid with a nauscating odour and used mainly as a strong purgative. Flower and leaves are also used to poison fishes. Seed dust is a strong and safe piscicide. The amount of dust recommended is 50-60 kg/hac. at 1 m. water depth. The seed dust poisonous effect remain for 3-5 days.

Euphorbia antiquorum (Tesiramansa, Euphorbiaceae) : Erect fleshy glabrous shrub or small tree. It is a common hedge plant with fleshy 3-angle stem and is naturalised in the village shrubberies. Milky latex-resin causes blindness.

Euphorbia hirta (Khirai, Euphorbiaceae) : Very small prostrate weed. Reported to be poisonous.

Jatropha gossypifolia (Lal-bharanda, Euphorbiaceae): This is a common shrub on roadsides or hedges. Reported to be poisonous.

Sesbania sesban (Joyanti, Leguminosae) : Common in the red soil of the west rardh. The freshly crushed stem bark is thrown in deep stagnant water to stupefy fish before catching. This mechanism is commonly used by the local fishermen.

Barringtonia acutangula (Hijal, Lecythidaceae) : Known locally as Hijal, it is common in lower Bengal and other parts of India. Much branched moderate tree. The bark is used in tanning. The bark is thrown in water to stupefy fish before catching (Chakrabarty *et al.* 1972). About 150 kg/hac. of bark and seed dust at 1 meter depth kills the fishes. The toxic effect initiates within two hours and lasts between 3 and 4 days.

Acacia concinna (Bon rita, Mimosaceae) : Twinning shrub, sometimes grown on the village thickets and roadside hedges. Pods contain saponin which is toxic.

Melia azedarach (Maha neem, Meliaceae) : Large deciduous tree which is larger than Neem. Planted as an avenue tree. Seed dust acts as piscicides by causing nervous disorder. A dosage of 2000 kg/hac. in water is sufficient to kill the aquatic fauna within 2 to 5 hrs. The poisonous effect persist for 25-35 days.

Melia azadirachta (Neem, Meliaceae) : Medium tree, commonly found in village surrounding, roadsides and in forests. Possesses bitter taste in bark and leaves. Fruits contains azadirachtin which has toxic effects.

Abrus precatorius (Kunch, Papilionaceae) : Found generally on the forest-bushes or climbing over the tree on the waste lands. Seeds are red, a black round spot (black eye) is present on the seed. Seed powder contains abrin which is highly toxic and soluble in salt water.

Derris indica (Karanjo, Papilionaceae) : Medium tree, found near hedges, waste lands, roadsides and railway tracksides. Seed dust acts as piscicides and insecticides and oil is very useful.

Derris scandens (Noalota, Papilionaceae) : Large climber, very common on forest-bushes (near the scrub-jungles). Its roots contain very poisonous rotenone which inhibits the cellular respiration of the fishes. Root powder of 100-150 kg/hac. at 1 m. depth is used for killing the fishes and the toxic effect lasts for 12-15 days. *Derris* plants were first used as fish toxicant prior to 1834 in Michigan.

Rhynchosia minima (Papilionaceae) : Annual herb. Seed powder is reported toxic to the fishes.

Clematis gouriana (Chhagalboti, Ranunculaceae) : A shrub which climbs by twisting the petiole. Strong acrid, toxic used as piscicide.

Tephrosia candida (Papilionaceae) : Generally found in the wet places. The leaves and bark are used as piscicides.

Polygonum hydropiper (Pakur mul, Polygonaceae) : Annual herb, a common weed of damp places. Commonly found on the margins of ponds, canal-ditches and roadsides. Plant juice is poisonous to fishes.

Nauclea orientalis (Rubiaceae) : Small tree with bushy crown. The bark powder is poisonous to the fish.

Madhuca indica (Mahua, Sapotaceae) : A large deciduous tree, occasionally planted and frequently found in Joypur, Sonamukhi forest. Mahua oil is a strong poison to fishes and also act as fish toxicant for removal of unwanted fishes and predators. Within 10-15 days, the decomposed oil cakes serve as a good manure to the fish ponds.

Pterospermum suberifolium (Muchkunda, Sterculiaceae) : Large tree, sometime found in roadsides and jungles. The wood is red, green fruits take an year for ripening. The flower and fruits are reported to be poisonous to insects (bed-bug) and to the fishes.

Nicotiana tabacum (Tamak, Solanaceae) : A small shrub with sticky glandular hair, grown in all climate conditions throughout the year in a well-drained light and sandy loam. Nicotine is the chief alkaloid and is present higher quantities (2-5%) in leaves than other plant parts. The alkaloid bears neurotoxic effect. Dry leaf dust is sufficient to kill the fishes and other aquatic fauna. Toxicogenic effect of nicotine last for 3-4 days after which the zooplanktons begin to reappear.

Nicotiana rustica (Hookah tamak, Solanaceae) : It is a smaller plant, cultivated during cool weather and mainly grown as a rotation crop with maize and groundnut in alluvial soils. Dry leaf dust acts as piscicides.

Cleome viscosum (Ghetu, Verbenaceae) : Robust shrub found in waste lands and contains clerodin which is sufficient to kill within 30 minutes the earthworms and tiny fishes.

Clerodendrum infortunatum (Ghetu, Verbenaceae) : Shrub found in the waste lands, roadsides and the plant contain clerodin and oleic acid which is toxic to fishes.

4 DEFINITIONS OF SOME TERMS

Ethno Botany- It is a branch of botany that focuses on plant that injure, heal and nourish or alter the conscious mind by Folk doctors.

Abortifacient- Anything used to cause or induce abortion.

Abscess- A localized collection of pus in any part of the body.

Allergy- (Gr, allos, other, ergon, work). It is a condition of hypersensitivity of the body cells to specific substances resulting various types of reactions.

Analeptic- The agent that excites and stimulates and causes generalised convulsions.

Angiodema- It is a condition of temporary swelling of skin associated with urticaria and crythema.

Anthrax- Acute, infectious disease caused by *Bacillus anthracis.* Usually attacking cattle, horses and sheeps.

Antidote- A substance that neutralizes poisons or their effect.

Antiseptic- An agent capable of producing antisepsois.

Aphrodisiac- A drug which promotes sexual desire.

Asthma- A disease of the bronchial tube causing recurrent attacks of breathlessness and coughing.

Ayurvedic Medicine- This is a branch of medicine based on the Hindu scriptures or Vedas. This type is considered as indigenous Indian system of medicine.

Carminative- A drug which relieves flatulence.

Compound System- The enzymatic system that is activated by antigen-antibody reactions to act sequentially and to activate and amplify the activity of successive components thus affecting chemotaxis, bacteriolysis. The enzymatic system is composed of 9 separate components (C_1 - C_9) and 11 serum proteins.

Dandruff - Normal exfoliation of the epidermis of the scalp in the form of dry white scales.

Depressant- These are the agents that reduces functional activity.

Dermatitis- This may be defined as a condition where inflammation of the skin is observed.

Diaphoretic- This is a condition which promotes perspiration.

Diplopia- This is referred when the vision is double.

Diuretic- The agent that increases urine flow is known as diuretic.

Dysmenorrhoea- Pain in association with menstruation.

Dysuria- Painful and difficult urination.

Eczema- Itching skin disease.

Edema- This is a condition where abnormal accumulation of fluid between the cells takes place.

Emetic- The agent that induces vomiting.

Epilepsy- This is a condition where disorder characterized by severe muscular spasms.

Ergotism- This is a kind of disease showing spasms, cramps and various cerebrospinal disorders due to excessive use of medicinal ergot or of eating ergot containing grains.

Flatulence - Excessive gas in the stomach and intestines.

Freckles- Coloured spots on the exposed parts of the skin.

Galactagogue- An agent that promotes the secretion and flow of milk.

Haematuria- Passing of blood in the urine.

Lathyrism- This is a kind of disease showing spastic paralegia, pain, hyperesthesia and parathesia leading to death due to ingestion of seeds of a leguminoceous species Lathyrus.

Leucoderma- A skin disease marked by skin losing its pigment partially or wholly.

Menorrhagia- Abnormally excessive menstruation.

Myxedema- This is a kind of disorder that is hypothyroid induced and this is characterized by dry waxy skin due to mucin deposits.

Narcotic- A drug which induces deep sleep or insensibility to pain.

Nephritis- Inflammation of the kidneys.

Neuroleptic- This is tranquilizing agent, generally without hypnotic affect. This is generally observed as psychomotor activity.

Peristalsis- It is an action where rhythmatic contraction and relaxation along the intestine promoting movement of contents.

Pharmacognosy- The study of natural drugs and their natural constituents is known as pharmacognosy.

Photodermatitis - This is inflammation of skin resulting from activation by light of chemicals on the skin.

Phytohemagglutinin (PHA) - It is a plant product, mitogenic lectin that agglutinates erythrocytes and stimulates thymus-derived lymphocytes.

Pyorrhoea - A purulent discharge from the gums.

Pyretic - It is referred to a kind of fever.

Rheumatic Fever - This is a kind of fever due to inflammation of heart fibrous tissue leading to scarring of heart valves and the joints; occurs as an immunological sequel to *Streptococcus pyrogens* infection elsewhere.

Schizophrenia - This is a mental disease that involves the disorganization of personality and characterized by delusions, hallucination, abnormal behaviour and retreat from reality.

Sedative - An agent used to relieve tension and anxiety.

Styptic - An agent which checks bleeding.

Suppuration - The process of pus formation.

Synesthesia - It is a condition in which a stimulus of one sense is perceived as sensation of a different sense.

Thrush - It is due to infection by *Candida* sp. (Fungi Imperfecti) of oral mucous membranes, usually in childhood.

Toxicomania - This is referred to periodic or chronic state of intoxication as a result of repeated use of a drug harmful to the individual or society.

Ulcer - An open sore on the skin or mucous membrane.

Unani Medicine - This is branch of medical science that are based on traditional medical system found in the Muslim world.

Vermifuge - A drug which expels intestinal worms.

Wheal and Flare - The immediate response to histamine release or other minor nonpenetrating injuiry to the skin is known as wheal and flare. This is followed by wheal or edema radiating from the line of injury. It is considered as a characteristic skin lesion of immediate hypersensitivity.

Zoopharmacognosy- Animal's self medication.

5

Amusing Common Names of Some Plants

Name literally means a word by which a person, a plant, an animal, a place or a thing is known or indicated. A name is gained due to one's features, activities, appearance, relation with others, a myth or a local belief. Plants are no exception. Poor man's beef stick *(Fistulina hepatica)* is called so due to its appearance as that of beef and when broken a blood like red exudates oozes out of its body. *Trapa bicornata* fruit has two thorns and resembles head of a bull and is called 'bull's head'. 'Lovage' *(Levisticum officinale)* has got its name due to the belief that its leaves are eaten to feel like making love.

Certain local names are appearing because they are amusing. Following is a brief list of plants with their common amusing names:

Local Names	Botanical Names	Common Names	Family
Kunch	*Abrus precatorius*	Carb's eye	Leguminosae
	Acetabularia sp.	Mermaid's wine glass	Dasycladaceae
	Aframomum melegueta	Grain of paradise	Zingiberaceae
	Alchemilla vulgaris	Lady's mantle	Rosaceae
Chatim	*Alstonia scholaris*	Devil tree	Apocynaceae
	Amaranthus sp.	Love-lies-bleeding	Amaranthaceae
	Amaranthus sp.	Joseph's coat	Amaranthaceae
	Amaranthus cruentus	Prince's feather	Amaranthaceae
Ata/Nona	*Annona reticulata*	Bullock's heart	Annonaceae
	Anthyllis barba-jovis	Jupiter's beard	Leguminosae
	Araucaria araucana	Monkey puzzle	Araucariaceae
	Arisaema speciosum	Snake or cobra plant	Araceae
	A.triphyllum	Jack-in-the-pulpit	Araceae
	Auricularia auricula-judae	Jew's ear	Phargmobasidiomycetes

contd...

Local Names	Botanical Names	Common Names	Family
Raktokanchan	*Bauhinia variegata*	Camel's foot trace	Leguminosae
	Brassica oleracea var. germmifera	Brussels sprout	Brassicaceae
	Brunfelsia americana	Lady-of-the-night	Solanaceae
	Capsella bursa-pastoris	Shepherd's purse	Brassicaceae
	Castilleja sp.	Painted lady, paint brush	Scrophula-riaceae
Jhau	*Casuarina equisetifolia*	Beef wood tree	Casuarinaceae
	Celosia cristata	Cook's comb	Amaranthaceae
Morogjhuti	*Ceratonia silliqua*	St. John's bread	Leguminosae
Hasnahana	*Cestrum nocturnum*	Queen of the night	Solanaceae
	Chelone Sp.	Turflehead	Scrophula-riaceae
Chor-Kanta	*Chrysopogon aciculatus*	Love thorn	Gramineae
Bathua	*Chenopodium album*	Goose-foot	Chenopodi-aceae
Amrah	*Spondias pinnata*	Hog-plum	Anacardiaceae
Bamunhati	*Clerodendrum indicum*	Turk's turban	Verbenaceae
	Clerodenron thomasonae	Bleading heart	Verbenaceae
Kalo-Kunch	*Coix lachryma-jobi*	Job's tears	Gramineae
Colchicin	*Colchicum autumnale*	Naked lady	Liliaceae
	Convallaria majalis	Lily of the Valley	Liliaceae
	Cynoglossum officinale	Forget-me-not, Hound's tongue	Boraginaceae
	Entada gigas	Nicker-bean	Leguminosae
	Euphorbia sp.	Mother-in-laws tongue	Euphorbiaceae
	E.marginata	Snow on the mountains	Euphorbiaceae
	E.splendens	Crown of thorns	Euphorbiaceae
	Fistulina hepatica	Ox tongue, Poor man's beef-stick	Polyporaceae
	Ginko biloba	Maiden hair	Ginkgoaceae
Dhenras	*Hibiscus esculentus*	Ladie's finger	Malvaceae
	Ipomoea cornea	The bush that flies	Convolvulaceae
	Iresine sp.	Blood leaf, Juba's bush	Amaranthaceae
	Lappula dellexa	Beggar's lice	Boraginaceae
	Levisticum officinale	Lovage	Umbelliferaceae
Kayet bel	*Limonia acidissima*	Elephant apple	Rutaceae
	Linaria vulgaria	Toad flax, Butter-and-eggs	Scrophulari-aceae

contd...

Local Names	*Botanical Names*	*Common Names*	*Family*
Parol	*Luffa cylindrica*	Bath sponge	Cucurbitaceae
Baghnokh	*Martynia annua*	Tiger's nail	Martyniaceae
Lajjabati	*Mimosa pudica*	Touch-me-not	Mimosaceae
	Mimulus luteus	Monkey flower	Scrophulariaceae
Sandhyamoni	*Mirabilis jalapa*	Four O'clock plant, Marvel of Peru	Nyctaginaceae
Sajina	*Moringa oleifera*	Drumstick, horse radish	Moringaceae
Kamini	*Murraya paniculata*	Chinese box	Rutaceae
	Mysotis arvensis	Forget-me-not	Boraginaceae
	Nigella damascena	Love-in-a-mist	Ranunculaceae
Kalo-tulsi	*Ocimum sanctum*	Sacred basil	Labiatae
	Oxalis repens	Wood-sorrel	Oxalidaceae
Jhumkalata	*Passiflora foetida*	Passion flower	Passifloraceae
Tentule sirish	*Pithecolobium saman*	Rain tree	Leguminosae
Gulancha	*Plumeria rubra*	Temple tree	Apocynaceae
Jhinga	*Luffa acutangula*	Ridge gourd	Cucurbitaceae
Chichinga	*Trichosanthes anguina*	Snake gourd	Cucurbitaceae
Karala	*Momordica charantia*	Bitter gourd	Cucurbitaceae
Lau	*Lagenaria siceraria*	Bottle gourd	Cucurbitaceae
Begun	*Solanum melongena*	Egg plant	Solanaceae
Alu	*S.tuberosum*	Apple of the earth	Solanaceae
Palash	*Butea frondosa*	Flame of the forest Bastard-teak	Papilionaceae
Pani-phal	*Trapa bicornata* (T. bispinosa)	Bull's head	Hydrocaryaceae
Siris	*Albizia lebbeck*	Parrot tree	Mimosaceae
Kachu	*Colocasia esculenta*	Elephant ear	Araceae
Arhar	*Cajanas cajan*	Pigeon pea	Papilionaceae
Barbati	*Vigna sinensis*	Cow pea	Papilionaceae
Bel	*Aegle marmelos*	Wood-apple	Rutaceae
Dhutura	*Datura metel*	Thorn-apple	Solanaceae
Ophioglossum	*Ophioglossum vulgatum*	Adder's tongue fern	Ophioglossaceae
Chalta	*Dillenia indica*	Elephant apple	Dilleniaceae
Khejur	*Phoenix dactylifera*	Date palm	Palmae
Kagzi lebu	*Cirtus aurantifolia*	Lime	Rutaceae
Bancharal	*Desmodium gyrans*	Telegraph plant	Papilionaceae
	Polyporus mylitae	Blackfellow's bread	Polyporaceae

6

REFERENCES

Bodding, P.O. 1927. Studies in Santal medicine and connected folklore-II. Santal medicine, Mem. Asiat. Soc. Bengal. 10:133-426.

Chakraborty, D.P., Nandy, A.C. and Philligose, M.T. 1972. *Barringtonia acutangula* L. Gaertn as fish poison. Indian J. Exptl. Biol. 10:78-80.

Chaudhuri, R.H.N., Saren, A.M. and Molla, H.A. 1982. Some less known uses of plants from the tribal areas of Bankura district, West Bengal. Indian Mus. Bull. 14:71-73.

Chopra, R.N., Nayar, S.L. and Chopra, I.C. 1956. Glossary of Indian Medicinal Plants, C.S.I.R., New Delhi.

Chopra, R.N., Chopra, I.C., Handa, K.L. and Kapur, L.D. 1958. Chopra's indigenous drugs of India. Calcutta. U.N. Dhar and Sons Pvt. Ltd.

Chopra, R.N., Chopra, I.C. and Verma, B.S. 1969. Supplement to Glossary of Indian Medicinal Plants. C.S.I.R., New Delhi.

Ghosh, A., Maity, S. and Maity, M. 1996. Ethnomedicine in Bankura district, West Bengal. J. Econ. Taxon. Bot. Addl. Series. 12:318-320.

Ghosh, A. 1999. Herbal veterinary medicine from the tribal areas of Bankura district. J.Econ. Taxon. Bot. 23:557-560.

Ghosh, A. 2002. Herbal veterinary medicine from the tribal areas of Bankura and Midnapur district. In: Series Recent Progress in Medicinal Plants. Vol. 1. Ethnomedicine and Pharmacognosy (Eds:V.K. Singh, J.N. Govil and Gurdip Singh). Sci Tech. Pub., USA.pp. 233-237.

Jain, S.K. 1965, Medicinal plantlore of the tribals of the Bastar. Econ. Bot. 19: 236-250.

Jain, S.K. 1968. Medicinal plants. National Book Trust, New Delhi.

Jain, S.K. 1981. Glimpses of Indian Ethnobotany. Oxford and IBH Publishing company, New Delhi.

Jain, S.K. and Banerjee, D.K. 1974. Preliminary observations on the ethnobotany of the genus *Coix*. Econ. Bot. 28:38-42.

Jain, S.K. and Rao, R.R. 1976. A hand book of field and herbarium methods. Today and Tomorrow Pub., New Delhi.

Jain, S.K. and Tarafdar, C.R. 1970. Medicinal Plantlore of the Santals. Econ. Bot. 24: 241-278.

Kirtikar, K.R. and Basu, B.D. 1975. Indian Medicinal Plants. Vols.1 and 2. Bishen Singh Mahendra Pal Singh, Dehra Dun.

Mudgal, V. 1987. A manual of Ethnobotany (Ed: S.K. Jain). Scientific Publishers, Jodhpur. pp 58-68.

Mukherjee, A and Namhata, D. 1988. Herbal veterinary medicine as practised by the tribals of Bankura district, West Bengal. J. Bengal Natural History Society, 7 : 69-71.

Namhata, D. and Mukherjee, A 1988. Ethnomedicine in Bankura district, West Bengal. Indian J. Applied and Pure Biol. 2:53-55.

Namhata, D. and Ghosh, A 1993. Herbal folk medicine of Bankura district, West Bengal. Geobios new reports. 12: 94-96.

Naskar, K.R. 1986. Trends of aquatic weed management through proper utilization. Proc. Nat. Sem. Recent Trend in Plant Sci. Res., Santiniketan.

Naskar, K.R. and Guha Bakshi, D.N. 1987. Mangrove swamps of the Sunderban. An Ecological perspective. Naya Prakash, Calcutta.

Pal, D.C. 2002. Lodha Medicine of Midnapore district, West Bengal. In: Series Recent Progress in Medicinal plants. Vol.7. Ethnomedicine and Pharmacognosy II (Eds. V.K. Singh, J.N. Govil, Shamima Hashmi and Gurdip Singh). Sci. Tech. Pub. USA. pp. 443-464.

Perry, L.M. 1980. Medicinal plants of east and southeast Asia. MIT, Cambridge, MA. Wealth of India (Raw materials). 1948-1976. CSIR, New Delhi.

Singh, U., Wadhwani, A.M. and Johri, B.M. 1988. Dictionary of Economic Plants in India. I.C.A.R., New Delhi.

Tyler, E. Varro, Lynn R., Brady, James Robbers. 1981. Pharmacognosy, 8th Edition, USA.

Wealth of India (Raw materials). 1948-1976. CSIR, New Delhi.

7

List of Publications by Author in East & West

1. J. Agronomy & Crop Science 162, 342-346 (1989). Paul Parey Scientific Publishers. Berlin and Hamburg ISSN 0931-2250. Monocarpic Senescence in Relation to Yielf of *Sesamum indicum* during source – Sink Alteration, A.K. Biswas and A.K. Ghosh.
2. *Indian J. Plant Physiol.*, Vol. XXXII, No. 2. pp. 172-174 (June, 1989). Monocarpic Senescence of *Arachis hypogaea* : Nutrient Withdrawal vs. Migration of Senescence Signal. A.K Ghosh and A.K. Biswas.
3. Indian Journal of Experimental Biology, Vol. 28, May 1990. pp. 492-493. Whole plant senescence in *Ophioglossum vulgatum* : Influence of sporangiferous spike, kinetin and abscisic acid. Arun Kumar Biswas, Ashis Kumar Ghosh, Swapan Kumar Mandal & Udayan Sarkar.
4. *Indian J. Plant Physiol.*, Vol. XXXIV, No. 1, pp. 25-29 (March, 1991). Source – Sink Relationship during Ageing and Senescence of *Solanum tuberosum* L. A.K. Ghosh and A.K. Biswas.
5. Agri. Biol. Res. 7(2) 132-138 (1991). Source – Sink Relationship during Monocarpic Senescence of *Raphanus sativus*. A.K. Ghosh and A. Biswas.
6. Indian Journal of Forestry Vol. 16(3) : 201-203. 1993. Intact Leaf Senescence in Some Polycarpic Forest Trees in Relation to their Reproductive Development. A.K. Ghosh and A.K. Biswas.
7. *Geobios new Reports 12* : 94-96, 1993. Herbal Folk Medicines of Bankura District, West Bengal. D. Namhata and A. Ghosh.
8. *Geobios new Reports 12* : 96-99, 1993. Effect of Polluted Air of Durgapur on the Vegetation. A.K. Ghosh.
9. *Revista Biol (Lisboa) 15* : 63-68, 1994. Monocarpic Senescence in *Amaranthus tricolour* L. : Dual Action of Kinetin. A.K. Ghosh and A.K. Biswas.
10. Indian Journal of Experimental Biology. Vol. 32. November, 1994, pp. 807-811. Correlative senescence in *Tagetes patula and*

Chtysanthemum coronarium during reproductive development. A.K. Ghosh and A.K. Biswas.

11. J. Agronomy & Crop Science 175-202 (1995). Blackwell Vissenshafts Verlag, Berlin ISSN 0931-2250. Regulation of Correlative Senescence in *Arachis hypogaea* L. by Source – Sink Alteration through Physical and Hormonal Means. A.K. Ghosh and A.K. Biswas.
12. J. Econ. Taxon. Bot. Additional Series, 12. Scientific Publishers, Jodhpur (India), 1996, pp. 318-320. Ethnomedicine in Bankura district, West Bengal. A.K. Ghosh, S. Maity and M. Maity.
13. Fifth West Bengal State Science Congress held at University of North Bengal, March 21-23, 1998. Herbal Veterinary medicine from the Tribal Area of Bankura District, West Bengal, A.K. Ghosh.
14. The Botanica, Vol. 42, pp. 20-23 (1993). Magazine of Delhi University Botanical Society, Inhibitory Effect of Fishes Exposed to some Cultivated, Wild Plants from the Bangiya West Rardh (Bankura district), A.K. Ghosh.
15. Pak. J. Sci. Ind. Res. 2002, 45(3) : 212. Mechanism of Monocarpic Senescence of *Trichosanthes dioica* Roxb. (Cucurbitaceae), A.K. Ghosh.
16. Ghosh A.K. (2002). "Herbal Veterinary Medicine from the Tribal Areas of Bankura and Midnapur District". In : Series Recent Progress in Medicinal Plants. Vol. 1 – Ethnomedicine & Pharmacognosy (Eds : V.K. Singh, J.N. Govil and Gurdip Singh). Sci. Tech. Pub., USA, 233-237.
17. Indian Journal of Traditional Knowledge, Vol. 1 (i) October, 2002, pp. 93-95. Ethnoveterinary medicines from the tribal areas of Bankura and Medinipur districts, West Bengal. A. Ghosh.
18. J. Econ. Taxon. Bot. Vol. 27 No. 3 (2003). Scientific Publishers (India), pp. 573-575. Herbal veterinary medicine from the tribal areas of Midnapur & Bankura district, West Bengal, A.K. Ghosh.
19. J. Econ. Taxon. Bot. Vol. 27 No. 4 (2003), Scientific Publishers (India), pp. 825-826. Traditional Vegetable dyes from Central West Bengal. A. Ghosh.
20. Indian Journal of Traditional Knowledge, Vol. 2(4) October 2003, pp. 393-396. Herbal Folk Remedies of Bankura and Medinipur districts, West Bengal. A. Ghosh.
21. Natural Product Radiance Vol. 3(2), p. 91, March-April, 2004. Plant and Clay dyes used by Weavers and Potters in West Bengal. A. Ghosh.

22. Natural Product Radiance Vol. 3(3), p. 170, May-June 2004. Apiphilic plants in Agro-forestry. A. Ghosh.
23. Natural Product Radiance Vol. 3(3), p. 173, May-June 2004. Natural Biocides and Biofertilizers, A. Ghosh.
24. Natural Product Radiance Vol. 3(6), p. 426, Nov.-Dec. 2004. Home Made Baby Food. A. Ghosh and J. Karan.
25. Pak. J. Sci. Ind. Res. 2005, 48(1) : 55-56. Mechanism of Monocarpic Senescence of *Momordica dioica* : Source – Sink Regulation by Reproductive Organs, A. Ghosh.
26. Non-wood News, No. 12, p. 30, March 2005. Rome, Italy, Plant and Clay Dyes. A. Ghosh.
27. Ageing and Society : The Indian Journal of Gerontology, Vol. 15 (3 & 4), pp. 75-81, 2005. How one can survive for a long time in the earth. A. Ghosh.
28. Ghosh A. (2004). Identification of Veterinary Medicinal Plants through Participatory Approach. In : Advances in Medicinal Plants (Eds. N.D. Prajapati, T. Prajapati & S. Jajpura) Vol. 2, pp. 97-105. Asian Medicinal Plants and Health Care Trust, Jodhpur, Rajasthan.
29. Natural Product Radiance, Vol. 5 (4), p. 260. July-Aug. 2006. Healthy Pan-drink. A. Ghosh.
30. J. Econ. Taxon. Bot. Vol. 30 (Suppl.), pp. 233-238. (2006). Medicinal plants used for treatment of diabetes by the tribals of Bankura, Purulia and Medinipur of West Bengal. A. Ghosh.
31. Natural Product Radiance, Vol. Ethnobotanical Survey in West Rarrh of Natural Health and Green Belt Movement. A. Ghosh.

Books

1. Regulation of Senescence in Various Plants by A.K. Biswas & A.K. Ghosh, Emkay Publications, Delhi.
2. Paribesh O Udvid, A. Ghosh.
3. Prani Rahasya, A. Ghosh.
4. Ethnobiology : Therapeutics & Natural Resources, A. Ghosh, Daya Publishing House, New Delhi.
5. Ethnomedicine for Human and Veterinary Development, A. Ghosh, Daya Publishing House, New Delhi.

8
INDEX

8.1 PLANT INDEX

8.2 DISEASE INDEX

K

L

M

N

P

R

S